TREATING EPILEPSY NATURALLY

A GUIDE TO ALTERNATIVE

AND ADJUNCT THERAPIES

PATRICIA A. MURPHY

FOREWORD BY RUSSELL L. BLAYLOCK, M.D.

New York Chicago San Francisco Lisbon London Madrid Mexico City
Milan New Delhi San Juan Seoul Singapore Sydney Toronto

Library of Congress Cataloging-in-Publication Data

Murphy, Patricia A., 1951–
    Treating epilepsy naturally : a guide to alternative and adjunct therapies /
Patricia A. Murphy.
        p.   cm.
    Includes index.
    ISBN 0-658-01379-3
    1. Epilepsy—Alternative treatment.   2. Naturopathy.   I. Title.

RC372.M87   2001
616.8'53—dc21   2001029778

6 7 8 9 10 11 12 13 14 15 16 17 18 19 20 21   DOC/DOC   0 9 8 7

ISBN 978-0-658-01379-9
MHID   0-658-01379-3

Cover design by Bill Stanton/Stanton Design
Cover illustration by Kathy Obringer
Interior design by Jeanette Wojtyla

McGraw-Hill books are available at special quantity discounts to use as premiums and
sales promotions, or for use in corporate training programs. For more information, please
write to the Director of Special Sales, Professional Publishing, McGraw-Hill, Two Penn
Plaza, New York, NY 10121-2298. Or contact your local bookstore.

This book is printed on acid-free paper.

For Jesse Sinclair

Contents

PART III *Listening to Your Body*

PART IV *Age, Gender, and Epilepsy*

PART V *Creating a Supportive Environment*

FOREWORD ——————————————————

One of the most devastating and disturbing things that can beset a human being is the loss of control of one's nervous system. Author Pat Murphy tells us from firsthand experience what it is like to have your life torn apart by epilepsy.

References to epilepsy are found as far back as recorded human history. While there is no question that we have come very far in understanding the disorder, our treatment still leaves much to be desired. In all areas of medicine, I have observed an enormous gap between what we learn through our scientific studies and how we apply that knowledge. *Treating Epilepsy Naturally* provides the reader with a tremendous amount of scientific information concerning epilepsy, especially in the area of research that has remained untapped by conventional medicine.

Medical care has changed drastically over the past ten years. Patients, dissatisfied with how they are being treated by the medical profession, have decided to seek answers on their own. What we are finding is that in many cases the patients learn more about their disease than even the expert, a phenomenon that has been greatly enhanced by the Internet. Oftentimes when patients enter our offices, we find that they have already researched their illness and the lesser-known treatment options. They also know all about the medications that are being used along with their complications. With this base of knowledge patients have grown dissatisfied with the pat answers their physicians frequently give them. For example, when they ask about using a special nutritional supplement that research has shown to be helpful in their condition, they are often told, "There is no evidence that that works," or "That product can be dangerous and possibly interfere with your treatment."

What most patients don't know is that when their doctors make such statements, they often have no idea what they are talking about. In most cases they know little or nothing about the research concerning the use of the supplement and have little or no knowledge concerning the actual pathophysiology of the condition they are treating. Doctors in general have difficulty with biochemistry in medical school. Treatment of difficult-to-control conditions, such as epilepsy, requires an intimate knowledge of physiology and biochemistry. All medical conditions occur on a molecular level and involve numerous, often complex processes. If your doctors do not understand these molecular events, how can they efficiently treat your disorder?

In addition to this lack of knowledge, doctors often suffer from manipulation by their financiers. Most doctors are trained in medical universities that receive their major financing from pharmaceutical companies. As a result, they are oriented toward pharmaceutical treatment of diseases. Make no mistake, pharmaceutical drugs have made a major contribution to our health, but they have also created a whole new kind of disease, one that can be fatal, called *iatrogenic diseases*. These are disorders caused by the treatment itself. More than five hundred thousand people a year suffer major and even fatal complications from pharmaceutical drugs. In comparison, fewer than two hundred fifty thousand people suffer from complications from taking natural products, and most of these are minor.

Most physicians know little about alternative treatments and too often dissuade or discourage their patients from trying them. Therefore, it is important to do some research of your own. Should your doctor tell you some natural product is dangerous or ineffectual, ask him or her to provide you with the medical documentation to back it up. You can provide the scientific documentation you have found to support your use of the product and discuss this with your doctor.

This book approaches epilepsy from all aspects of the disorder: diet, supplements, exercise, sleep requirements, and stress reduction, as well as special nutraceuticals to reduce the risk of having further seizures. This comprehensive approach is vital in controlling such a devastating disorder because so many factors can affect the likelihood of having a seizure.

This book discusses one of my principal interests: excitotoxicity. Excitotoxicity is a central cause of numerous conditions affecting the nervous system, including viral encephalitis, neurological effects of Lyme disease, AIDS dementia, head trauma, Alzheimer's disease, Parkinson's disease, stroke, Huntington's disease, Lou Gehrig's disease, and epilepsy. There is a strong connection between excitotoxicity and free-radical injury within the affected parts of the brain in these disorders. This is why preventing exposure to excitotoxins, such as monosodium glutamate (MSG), hydrolyzed vegetable protein, aspartame, and natural flavoring, is so important for the epilepsy patient.

Most of the new pharmacological seizure medications are aimed at preventing this excitotoxic reaction in the seizure focus within the brain. Many natural products significantly reduce the excitotoxic process, thereby lowering the seizure risk. For example, magnesium and zinc, two elements strongly associated with reducing seizures, act to reduce the excitotoxin-triggered explosion of neuron activity we call a seizure.

This book also includes biofeedback control exercises that can regulate brain discharge activity. This is one of the beauties of the nervous system: its ability to control itself. The ability of the brain to control itself and its many connections to the body has led to a whole new discipline in medicine called *psychoneuroimmunology*. There is sufficient evidence that the biofeedback system can control neuron discharge within specific parts of the brain as well.

I recommend this book as a helpful guide to anyone suffering from seizures. Only by approaching the disorder in all its many aspects can it be brought under control. Even if you will not be able to stop all of your antiseizure medications, you should be able to significantly lower the dose so that you can lead a more healthful life, free of the many complications associated with these medications. Through dietary discipline and rigorous adherence to these principles you can meet success.

—*Russell L. Blaylock, M.D.*
director, Advance Nutritional Concepts,
and clinical assistant professor of
neurosurgery at University of
Mississippi Medical Center

PREFACE

People diagnosed with epilepsy often get mixed messages: on the one hand, physicians usually tell patients that seizures are caused by defective neurons in the brain; yet the same physicians insist that the only way to control seizures is through anticonvulsant medication or brain surgery. In other words, the problem lies *within* but the treatment lies *outside* of us. This leaves many people feeling powerless, bewildered, and frustrated.

Most doctors have no suggestions for patients who want to treat their seizures with alternative therapies. Indeed, physicians often denigrate alternative therapies as being "unproven" (never mind that a Government Accounting Office study found that only 20 percent of conventional medical treatments have actually undergone double-blind, placebo-controlled studies). Even though researchers know far more about epilepsy today, the medical profession continues to treat the disorder merely as a brain malfunction—ignoring the advice of eminent neurologist Wilder Penfield (1891–1976), who said, "One must treat the whole person."

We struggle with the shame of having a body that seems defective; thus, we feel defective. As we work to dispel myths surrounding epilepsy, we need to dispel one myth promulgated by the medical profession: that prescribed medication and/or brain surgery are the only effective ways to treat seizures.

Some years ago, I mentioned to the publicity director of a local epilepsy organization that a respected nutritionist was willing to give the annual lecture. The publicity director was enthusiastic at first, but after speaking with the director of the organization, she changed her mind. "I don't think it's a good idea," she said. "We don't want to give people false hope."

But there is nothing false about this: every day, people with epilepsy are using safe, effective alternative treatments—alone or in conjunction with prescribed medication—to reduce or eliminate seizures. Most of these treatments—some ancient, some new—have been backed by anecdotal and scientific research. All of them demand further study.

Over the years, I've been fortunate to come into contact with health professionals who treat epilepsy as more than a problem of overfiring neurons, who helped me improve my physical, emotional, and mental health. In my own experience, alternative treatments, such as nutrition, biofeedback, and acupuncture, along with counseling, have helped me to greatly reduce my seizures and medication and to understand and trust my body in a way I never did when I was using only medication.

This book describes how to incorporate a range of treatments into daily life. It also provides information for children, women, men, and the elderly, who all face special problems that are sometimes worsened by conventional drug therapy. Since one of the top complaints of people with epilepsy is the insensitivity of physicians, I've also included ways to work with health-care practioners, particularly in carrying out alternative treatments. I believe that those of us with epilepsy don't just want to control seizures, we want to have greater control of our health. We want the ability to make informed choices.

ACKNOWLEDGMENTS ───────

So many people helped me create this book, and space prevents me from mentioning them all. But I am especially grateful to Steve and Michelle Handwerker for their support in the early stages of this book and to Margaret Backenheimer, Jim Brown, and Elaine Weiss for critical editorial help. Rudy Shur's suggestions helped to make this a better book, and I appreciate the kindness and insight of my editors, Peter Hoffman, Linda Laucella, and Katherine Hinkebein. I also want to thank the National Epilepsy Library staff, especially Cecille Jach, for research assistance.

I've been fortunate to know health professionals who helped me improve my health. Su Chen-Lor, my acupuncturist, knew just what my body needed. Dr. Robert Fried taught me how to breathe. Dr. Max Rudansky was not only the first neurologist who actually listened to me but also the first to acknowledge the benefit of alternative treatments. And Stan Kull, my periodontist, arrived just in time.

Finally, I am grateful to Michael for his unflagging good humor.

PART I

The Hidden Disorder

A Monster Beside Myself
My Story

> *There is power inherent in committing yourself to the process of creating health in all levels of your life.*
>
> —CHRISTIANE NORTHRUP, M.D., AUTHOR OF
> *Women's Bodies, Women's Wisdom*

A few days before my twenty-first birthday, I had a tonic-clonic seizure (also called *grand mal*). My parents rushed me to the hospital, where I underwent tests for several days. I was either dying, I thought, or the doctors would tell me to quit trying to burn the candle at both ends.

But no, I had *epilepsy.* I could hardly get the word past my lips. A hospital neurologist explained that tests showed an abnormal electrical discharge emanating from my brain. He said that if brain cells, part of a network of billions of cells continuously firing harmoniously, are overstressed, their discharge may recruit other cells and start a seizure. "Like a fuse blowing," he said.

Other than possible scar tissue formed after falling off a horse when I was fifteen, there didn't seem to be any external cause for the seizure, which meant I had *idiopathic* epilepsy. The neurologist seemed confident that the anticonvulsant medications he prescribed would prevent any more seizures from occurring. In other words, I needed to be protected from my own body.

Just as that doctor did, I saw epilepsy as something to be conquered, subdued. I dutifully took my medications, phenobarbital and Dilantin, every day. I carried a medical alert card. I read pamphlets published by the Epilepsy Foundation of America that tried to be informative and reassuring. They estimated that one or two out of every one hundred Americans had epilepsy.

Epilepsy was defined as a condition in which a person has recurrent seizures, which are temporary changes in behavior or activity brought on by excessive electrical discharges in the brain. Although tonic-clonic seizures are the type most closely associated with epilepsy, there are several different types of seizures.

Reading the descriptions of *absence* seizures (also called *petit mals*), I realized I had experienced them since I was a kid. I thought everyone else had them too, so I never found them to be unusual. Each one was very brief, lasting anywhere from a fraction of a second to several seconds. An absence seizure felt like a hitch in thought. Or it could eclipse a thought. Sometimes I had the sensation that someone had been talking to me and I would realize I hadn't been listening.

I also remembered Liz, my best friend in high school. She had epilepsy, although I didn't know it until one day during an exam when one side of her body went rigid for several minutes. The next day she admitted she had epilepsy and took medication, but she didn't say much else, so I felt uncomfortable asking questions. When I saw her several years later, she was still taking medication and told me that her husband had called her a drug addict. In retaliation, she abruptly stopped taking her medication but then had a seizure in front of her young son. I thought it was stupid of her to stop taking medication because of her husband's ignorance and cruelty. But now I recognize the self-hatred and anger that come from feeling you have to keep secrets about a body you occupy, a body you and others perceive as so hopelessly damaged that the only thing keeping you upright are the chemicals in those pills. Your sense of control comes from brightly colored pills.

The Dilantin and phenobarbital I took did control my seizures. In six years, I had just three seizures. But I paid a price for that control. My memory seemed slower, my coordination was off—sometimes a drinking glass would suddenly slip out of my hand—and I woke up groggy in the morning. While I had never felt very strong physically, now I felt downright fragile. But the biggest price I paid was shame. If anyone asked about the pills I took, I mumbled something about a neurological disorder. I never told employers I had epilepsy. I never discussed "it" with my family—just as we didn't discuss my mother's migraines or my father's heart problems. We were just victims.

Sometimes we're seeking something and don't even realize it; somehow, we're a step ahead of ourselves. Six years after my diagnosis, I went to a holistic health center. Unable to lose weight, I was convinced I had a sluggish thyroid and sought an alternative to the thyroid medication my doctor had prescribed. But what the physician and nutritionist at the center told me, essentially, was, "There's nothing wrong with your thyroid. You just eat too much."

They seemed certain that my body's inability to absorb the huge amounts of refined sugar in my diet played a key role in my seizures. I was skeptical of these people who used the word *energy* like a mantra, who said my favorite foods (cookies, ice cream, roast beef) were loaded with toxins and poisons. Hadn't the neurologist said there was no reason for my seizures? But I listened.

The body, they explained, is an energy system. For good health, energy must flow unimpeded throughout the body. Blockages cause illness and malfunction. When I consumed substances of no nutritional value, such as sugar, white flour, and preservatives, they hung around, slowing the digestive process, blocking up my system, and creating toxins. In my case, these substances went to my head, helping to create seizures. They weakened my immune system as well. A glucose-tolerance test showed I had hypoglycemia, a result of my pancreas not being able to manufacture insulin fast enough to process all the sugary foods I loved. That meant that the steady supply of energy my body—particularly my brain—needed wasn't always available.

At first I was very defensive. Nobody likes to hear criticism of her cherished eating habits. But enough of what they said struck a resonant chord. Still, changing my eating habits was difficult. Very difficult. A typical lunch for me had been fruit yogurt, a candy bar, and diet soda, with cookies later on. Switching to a lunch of raw vegetables, tofu or cottage cheese, a piece of fruit, and perhaps a few whole-grain crackers was a big adjustment. Dinners consisting of more salad, broiled chicken or fish, and a baked potato seemed dull. I wrote in my journal, "Cottage cheese tastes like chalk. Plain yogurt is contemptible. Of course I take my body for granted. I want to do the least possible. My body's supposed to take care of itself, isn't it?"

Admittedly, I felt wholesome buying brown rice and organically grown cabbage in health-food stores with names like Earth's Delight and Garden of Eatin'. Though I cheated often, eating Oreo cookies and Snickers bars, I gradually shifted my cravings from Pepperidge Farm cookies and chocolate-chip ice cream to juice-sweetened, wheat-free cookies, ice cream made from rice or soy, and carob, a healthier substitute for chocolate.

Sometimes, as I was selecting a package of carob cookies or even just contemplating eating something sweet that my body couldn't handle just then, my kneecaps would buckle, my elbows would tremble, my shoulders would become uncomfortably hot. Instinctively I realized that, like a child, my body was saying, "*I don't want it.*" Even a whiff of sugar in bakeries could bring on an absence seizure. My body was talking to me. I began listening and learning from my reactions to honey, wheat, corn, and dairy products. Realizing how much better I felt when they were eliminated from my diet, it was obvious that I was allergic to many foods I had consumed regularly.

It was a turnaround to realize my health could be affected by my diet. If the day of my epilepsy diagnosis had shut me off to choice, this experience with food opened the floodgate. My perception of epilepsy slowly changed from it being a burden into it being a bodily condition I could integrate and control by my decisions. I took yoga classes. I started riding my bicycle to work. In the space of about a year, I lost over forty pounds (and kept it off). For the first time I could remember, I possessed a feeling of well-being.

The physician at the holistic health center discontinued the phenobarbital I was taking and prescribed herbal tinctures of skullcap and goldenseal. Without the phenobarbital, I felt, at first, like my neurons were standing on end, but I no longer felt groggy when I woke up in the morning. My memory improved. I felt more alert throughout the day and didn't need those after-dinner naps. My headaches stopped. I didn't catch the colds going around the office. I actually had color in my cheeks.

It was a paradox: I was taking less medication and my body was actually more vulnerable to seizures, but I felt more in control. Before, I was being controlled—by the medication, by family, friends, and doctors who thought they knew what was best for me. Nearly everyone I knew thought I was foolish to lower my drug dosage and focus on nutrition, herbs, and vitamin supplements. But they didn't know what it was like to always feel tired, to feel limited, to fear their body. Sure, part of me longed to just take the medication and eat all the junk I wanted. But I couldn't. I wouldn't. Now I felt stronger, more connected to myself. Drugs treated the symptoms of my seizures, but they didn't come close to addressing *why* I had seizures. Even my mother's physician told me, "Drugs are a poison. But you have to decide whether the poison of one drug is worse than the poison of the illness. It's called risk-benefit ratio."

Unfortunately, over the next few months, I had several seizures, most of them in my sleep. My family said, "That shows you need to take the medication to prevent seizures!" But I didn't see it that way. The seizures happened when I was overtired or had eaten a lot of sweets. That's when I fully realized how much I cheated myself when I binged on ice cream or chocolate chip cookies, even if they were sweetened with rice syrup or pear concentrate. To my system, that was still sugar overload.

For me, a seizure feels like my neurons have imploded and reassembled themselves. When I wake up from a seizure, I feel disoriented. My head aches. I struggle to remember what day it is. It takes me days to get my epicenter, my equilibrium, back. After a seizure I feel guilty, too, certain that anyone who knew about the seizure would condemn me and tell me something was wrong with my energy, my emotions; that I was somehow at fault; that I had willed the seizure to happen. I used to get furious when my mother would say, "You just had a seizure. Doesn't it stand to reason that you're going to have more?" Yet, if I hadn't had a seizure for a while, she'd hint that I was due for one. I couldn't win.

One of the seizures I had was at the mental health clinic where I worked as a secretary. That seizure led to an informal, invaluable discussion about my epilepsy with Marty, a staff therapist. I remain forever grateful for that talk and for Marty's compassion. I had never before discussed how I felt about my seizures with anyone except health professionals. While talking with Marty, I found myself describing my epilepsy as "a kind of nebulous monster beside me." I realized I still had a long way to go before accepting the twilight part of me that lost consciousness, thrashed, and writhed. That part wasn't beside me but within me. I thought of the poet Rainer Maria Rilke's statement that "perhaps all the dragons of our lives are princesses who are only waiting to see us once beautiful and brave. Perhaps everything terrible is in its deepest being something help-less that wants help from us."[1] I took another step along the journey toward accepting and understanding my "monster." My body kept teaching me.

A few years later I learned how to breathe. I was fortunate enough to participate in an experimental biofeedback project for people with idiopathic epilepsy. It was conducted at the International Center for the Disabled in New York City and supervised by Robert Fried, Ph.D., and Richard Carlton, M.D. Once a week I sat in a room that resembled the cockpit of an airplane with electrodes pasted onto my scalp, facing a screen with lines that recorded my breaths. I don't know what I did, but for those twenty minutes, I communicated with my brain. "It's learning," Dr. Fried said. "And no one knows how we learn. How do you memorize a poem? No one knows."

The idea was to make the two lines on the screen come together in rounded curves. I learned that I usually breathed in sips and gulps, but to make the lines on the screen come together, I needed to breathe deeply, into my abdomen, and get more oxygen into my brain in order to achieve *alpha*, or relaxed, alert brain waves. In the process I was also changing my blood biochemistry.

In a human being, Dr. Fried said, "There is no such thing as a disease of the liver or heart or brain. Illness always involves the entire body. It may have its origin and its main effect in a particular organ, but it is never localized to that organ. We believe that, for people with idiopathic epilepsy, a seizure is not a manifestation of a disturbance in the brain. We believe it is a manifestation of the body of the individual as a whole, that there are dramatic changes that are produced by stress to the body, and these stress effects ultimately filter down to alterations in the oxygen transport system of the blood and that somehow winds up affecting the brain."

Being a shallow breather put a lot of stress on my body. It meant oxygen was being distributed unevenly in my lungs. In my everyday life, I noticed that when I got tense, like when I was trying to solve a problem at work, or worried about missing the train home, I stopped breathing. Or I sipped the air. Watching the lines on the biofeedback screen and pushing air deep into my abdomen, I felt like I was pushing past deep-seated anger and tension. I practiced breathing deeply and slowly all the time, taking in oxygen and not quickly blowing off the carbon dioxide that takes out toxins. I was so pleased when I made the lines connect on the biofeedback screen.

After years of research, Dr. Fried told me, he and his colleagues had come to the conclusion that seizures were metabolical, not neurological. They had redefined the word *metabolical* and had narrowed the definition to "the way in which blood carries oxygen to the brain. We believe that a seizure is basically an attempt to correct the effect of stress on individuals in their blood biochemistry," he said. "We are trying to give individuals techniques that help them to prevent the degradation of the oxygen transport system that then requires the body to call upon a seizure to straighten everything out. Breath controls brain waves. It's the body's natural tranquilizer.

"No one knows what starts a seizure," he continued, "but there are theories, the most prominent being that the process begins with the neurons, that there are defective neurons in the brain that start the process. Another theory is that metabolic processes cause toxic conditions in the body and that these toxic conditions in some way get into the disturbance of the metabolism of cells in the brain." Seizures, it seemed, could be caused by an array of things: diet, oxygen distribution, brain lesions, and more.

"Generally speaking," he said, "the medical profession views seizures as a pathological process—if you have seizures, you have a disease. We view it as a regulatory process, like vomiting. The seizure plays an important role in the physiological ecology of the individual, and in a sense, it readjusts the individual's metabolism. It really is a mechanism that the body looks to as a last-ditch effort to regain physiological balance—homeostasis."

According to Dr. Fried's theory, my body's losing consciousness was not the same as losing control. If a seizure was a regulatory process, then my body was merely trying to protect itself, to protect me. How can you hate a body that is trying to protect you, not betray you?

Even though I spent six months getting biofeedback treatments and went thirteen months without a seizure, my family and most of my friends remained skeptical of all this. I remember trying to explain to my perplexed mother the "energy radiating from my solar plexus," how sometimes it felt like butterflies, other times it felt like there was a miniature sun inside me. And I got no support at all from my neurologist. To him, holistic treatment belonged in the same category as voodoo and alchemy.

During the next few years, I started acupuncture treatments and went into therapy. They worked in tandem: acupuncture, intended to help correct and balance my body's energies, helped me pay closer attention to my body and how I reacted. I realized how I had always put a lid on exerting my body—not surprising, after a lifetime of hearing, "Be careful! Watch out! Take it easy! Don't run, you might fall down and kill yourself," and of course, "Don't do anything that might cause a seizure." With a therapist, I began looking

at why I had also put a lid on asserting myself or expressing powerful emotions such as anger, frustration, or happiness. I felt nothing
I did would ever be good enough, that I would always fail, always
have low-paying jobs, and live with my mother the rest of my life.
Years earlier, I had accepted the notion that I could create good
health by changing my eating habits. Now I had to confront the possibility that I could take charge of my life and have control by direct-
ing my thoughts and energies in positive, fulfilling ways.

Since conventional medicine had been of no great help to me
in understanding or accepting my seizures or my body, I was, for several years, opposed to it. Drugs just put my body to sleep; they fed
into my shame. To me, herbs were good; drugs were bad. Naturopaths and chiropractors were enlighted; physicians were benighted.
Then one day I had a seizure while riding my bicycle to see my
mother, who was ill in a nursing home. I wound up in the emergency
room of the local hospital, where an intern asked me the usual questions: Are you taking any new medication? Any illegal drugs? How
much sleep did you get last night? Then he asked me if I was menstruating. Stunned, I said yes. He said that due to hormone fluctuations many women with epilepsy experience *catamenial* seizures
before or during their period, something neither my neurologist nor
my acupuncturist had ever mentioned to me.

When I got home, I checked the calendar where my mother
recorded my seizures—something that had always infuriated me—
against the monthly red Xs (my menstrual period) on my own calendar. Both of the two seizures I had had during the past year were
during my period. When I was menstruating, I usually gave myself
permission to gorge on the sweets I loved. So at a time when my
seizure threshold was lowered, I was eating foods that lowered it still
further! It's unfortunate that I had to wind up in the emergency
room to learn this, but I very much appreciated that intern's observations. Since then, I've been particularly careful about what I eat

during menstruation. As Dr. Max Rudansky, the neurologist I started seeing soon after that incident, said, "Vigilance affords a kind of protection."

I continue to learn about nutrition, about the interplay between body and mind, and about optimal health. I follow a mostly vegetarian diet. I've lost much of my craving for sweets. I've gone twenty-seven months without a seizure. My EEGs are now normal. I can tell people I have epilepsy without stumbling over the word. No guilt. No shame. It just is. When I told a new acquaintance about my experiences with biofeedback and acupuncture, he later said to a friend of mine, "Don't you think it was beautiful the way she spoke about having epilepsy? That takes a person who's got it together."

Well, I haven't quite got my act together yet. Sometimes, I still fear "the monster within." A day doesn't go by that I don't think about the possibility of having a seizure. I know I could lose consciousness before I draw my next breath. I remember the way my mother used to look at me whenever I left the house, as though she might never see me again; the way my partner looks at me if I so much as make an odd sound. If I'm ever late, friends worry that I've had a seizure. I strike a balance between caution and confidence.

We all take different paths to sustain ourselves. Each body has its own particular wisdom, and within our bodies lay enormous healing resources. As world-famous physician and philosopher Albert Schweitzer said, "It's supposed to be a professional secret, but I'll tell you anyway. We doctors do nothing. We only help and encourage the doctor within."

CHAPTER 2

Epilepsy
Historical Perspectives

> *Epilepsy is an illness of various shapes and horrible.*
> —Aretaeus, from *The Falling Sickness: A History from the Greeks to the Beginning of Modern Neurology* by O. Temkin

Anybody can have a seizure. According to the Epilepsy Foundation of America, about 10 percent of all people experience a seizure at some point in their lives. It's not uncommon, for example, for an infant running a high temperature to have a convulsion. Or for a pressured college student missing meals and getting little sleep to have a seizure. A seizure can be a response to stress, hypoxia (insufficient oxygen), poorly controlled diabetes, alcoholism, drugs, low blood sugar, food allergies, even heart problems. Though a single seizure may be the initial event indicating epilepsy, the occurrence of one seizure doesn't necessarily indicate epilepsy.

The Epilepsy Foundation of America estimates that one or two out of every one hundred persons have epilepsy. People who have epilepsy may also have other types of disabilities, such as mental retardation or cerebral palsy, but seizures aren't caused by these conditions. More people in the United States have epilepsy than have cystic fibrosis, multiple sclerosis, and muscular dystrophy combined.[1] And 125,000 more Americans develop epilepsy each year. Yet epilepsy has never been a high-profile illness. For centuries, people with epilepsy haven't just suffered from seizures, they've also had to endure humiliation and discrimination.

Centuries of Misunderstanding

The word *epilepsy* comes from the Greek word *epilepsia*, which means "to take hold of, to seize." To the ancient Greeks, epilepsy was a miraculous phenomenon. After all, "only the gods," write neurologists Ley Sander and Pam Thompson, "could knock down a person, strip him of his reason, make his body thrash around, and afterwards bring him round with no apparent ill effects."[2]

The earliest reference to epilepsy is on a tablet dating from 2000 B.C., found in the Persian Gulf region. A few centuries later, the Code of Hammurabi in Babylonia (present-day southeastern Iraq) stated that anyone who bought a slave who had a seizure within a month of purchase was entitled to return that slave. This practice was also recorded in Egypt, in about the third or fourth century A.D., and was the practice of American slaveholders as well.[3]

The ancient Greeks referred to epilepsy as "the sacred disease," believing that someone who suffered seizures was under demonic possession. But in the fifth century B.C., Hippocrates, the most famous Greek healer of his day, wrote:

> [Epilepsy] appears to me nowise more divine nor more sacred than other diseases, but has a natural cause from which it originates. Men regard its nature and cause as

divine from ignorance and wonder because it is not at all like to other diseases.[4]

Hippocrates's view was the exception for centuries. In medieval Europe, people with epilepsy were thought to be possessed by the devil or infested with spirits. Exorcisms were routine. Epileptics were often taken for werewolves or kept in hospitals so their breath wouldn't contaminate others, or their ashamed families sequestered them at home.[5] In Shakespeare's *King Lear*, one of the lords scolds Oswald, the treacherous attendant to Goneril, Lear's unloving daughter, with the phrase, "A plague on your epileptic visage!" thus providing an indication of the image of epilepsy during the Elizabethan period.

Epilepsy has also been linked with insanity and sexual practices. In seventeenth-century England, one-third of the people in Bedlam, the insane asylum for the poor, disabled, and unwanted, reportedly had epilepsy. Moreover, in 1866 Dr. Baker Brown, an English physician, published *On the Curability of Certain Forms of Insanity, Epilepsy, Catalepsy, and Hysteria in Females*, in which he advocated the removal of the clitoris as a remedy for masturbation and epilepsy. Even in the late 1800s, it was not uncommon for people to believe that masturbation caused epilepsy and that castration was the cure.

Superstition and Science

For centuries epilepsy was considered a religious curse. But by the middle of the nineteenth century, that began to change. Physicians started observing people while they had seizures and studied the brains of those with epilepsy after they died. John Hughlings Jackson, an eminent neurologist, attributed seizures to discharges of nerve tissue. "Calm and cold scientific observation is needed," he wrote. Jackson studied innumerable seizures, including those of his wife, who had epilepsy. Though he published many studies about her seizures, he never considered how his wife's seizures might have affected her sense of self-esteem or competence. Unfortunately, the protocol that Jackson created, says neurologist Oliver Sacks, is "deaf to anguish."[6]

Although conventional medicine debunked the theory that epilepsy was due to demonic possession and classified it as a brain disorder, people with epilepsy continued to suffer discrimination, ostracism, and punishment. For example, the United States didn't allow immigrants who had epilepsy to enter the country. In 1891, the first American "epilepsy colony" was constructed in Gallipollis, Ohio. Another one opened in Abilene, Texas, in 1904 and served as a test center for phenytoin, or Dilantin, in the 1920s. Like their counterparts in England, people with epilepsy were more likely to be put in mental institutions than those with other illnesses. In 1878, an investigation of the New Jersey Mental Asylum found that to distinguish the "fakers" from those who actually had epilepsy, attendants poured alcohol over epileptic persons and set them on fire.[7]

Research in recent decades has shown that children of women with epilepsy have a very slightly increased risk of also developing seizures. That is by no means the only way a person develops seizures; however, a hundred years ago it was widely believed that epilepsy was inherited. Legislatures everywhere responded by passing laws to isolate those with epilepsy. Trying to rid the country of epilepsy, many states forbade epileptics to marry. Some were involuntarily sterilized.

Because of the possibility of pregnancy, having sex with a person with epilepsy became an offense. In 1903, the Connecticut legislature passed a law that would sentence anyone caught having sex with an epileptic person under forty-five years of age to no less than three years in prison. Even Margaret Sanger, an early advocate of birth control and women's rights, believed epilepsy was inherited and that anyone with epilepsy should be sterilized. Even in 1956, eighteen U.S. states still had laws permitting the involuntary sterilization of those with epilepsy. Steve Fishman, author of *Bomb in the Brain*, writes, "I know epileptics who have been carted off to mental wards, drunk tanks, or jail as the result of seizures."[8] In 1981, Kurt Eichenwald, who later became a reporter for *The New York Times* was dismissed from college because he was having occasional seizures. As James Trostle wrote in his article "Social Aspects of Epilepsy," "Industrial cultures have replaced the social quarantines of earlier times with other rationalized bureaucratic sanctions."[9]

I relate all of this because I believe that each person with epilepsy is still affected by the suffering of those who have lived with epilepsy before us. Though practices in the past are now illegal, and organizations like the Epilepsy Foundation of America have worked diligently to dispel stereotypes, we still grapple with misconceptions and fears. Lots of people believe epilepsy is punishment for some wrongdoing. Some parents still think epilepsy is contagious and won't let their kids play with kids who have epilepsy. And many parents are disappointed when their grown children decide to marry someone who has epilepsy.

A lot of people assume that people with epilepsy are mentally handicapped or mentally ill. While it's true that a number of retarded people do have epilepsy, and that epilepsy may occur with disabilities such as cerebral palsy or autism, it's also true that intelligent, gifted persons such as Peter Ilych Tchaikovsky, Fyodor Dostoyevsky, Alfred Nobel, Julius Caesar, and *Alice in Wonderland* author Lewis Carroll all had epilepsy. Concert pianist Lorin Hollander and the late actress/model Margaux Hemingway are two contemporary celebrities who publicly disclosed their epilepsy, as has former congressman Tony Coelho.

People with epilepsy may actually be more artistic and imagi-native than the general population. ("What is the neurology of imag-ination?" asks writer Adrienne Richard.) But a person's talents and imagination can be overlooked because he or she has seizures. When everyone around them fears and focuses on the seizures, it is to the detriment of the epileptic person's health and well-being.

Tracey Campbell, a writer who has epilepsy, once remarked, "I think that I could say to someone that I was an epileptic nude blonde 42-D rocket scientist that cured cancer and people would just hear the word epilept**ICK** and nothing more." A friend who is epileptic and manic-depressive once told me, "You feel that your body is a mistake. You're treated for *what* you are, not *who* you are. People look at you like you're a time bomb about to go off."

Other Cultures and Cultural Issues

While Western culture has traditionally looked upon seizures as something demonic, tending to punish those who have seizures, not all cultures perceive epilepsy this way. Some cultures believe that seizures are the result of possession by an evil spirit, an angry ancestor spirit, or punishment for doing something taboo. For example, the Navajo reportedly believe that sibling incest produces tonic-clonic seizures. In other cultures, a person who has seizures is looked upon with an aura of distinction because they are believed to have the power to perceive things other people cannot. Having seizures sometimes indicates shamanistic powers, even the power to heal.

Many health beliefs from different cultures have common themes: natural forces, supernatural forces, and the imbalance between forces (such as balancing yin and yang). Treatments usually involve a variety of home remedies, including potions and herbs, along with healing rituals involving the entire community. Many ethnic communities have folk healers.

In her book *The Spirit Catches You and You Fall Down* author Anne Fadiman relates with great compassion the conflict between a Hmong family from northern Laos, who are recent immigrants to California, and the physicians who treat their baby daughter, Lia Lee, who has seizures. Lia Lee's parents believe, as do many indigenous peoples, that epilepsy is caused by soul loss. ("The spirit catches you and you fall down" is the Hmong term for epilepsy.) But American-trained doctors believe Lia's seizures are caused by an electrochemical storm inside her head. Misunderstandings abound because the Lees speak almost no English, interpreters are not always available, and Lia continues to have seizures as doctors keep changing her medications. In less than four years, the prescriptions or their dosage changed twenty-three times. Her medical chart eventually weighed more than thirteen pounds.

Lia Lee's parents, confused by the prescriptions and the evidence that the medications were actually hurting their daughter, clung to the rituals and beliefs of their ancestors. They fed Lia teas made from herbs they grew, occasionally performed animal sacrifices, and even took her to a shaman in Minnesota. To them, the medications were worse than the seizures. Fadiman writes:

> Trying to understand Lia and her family by reading her medical chart was like deconstructing a love sonnet by reducing it to a series of syllogisms. Every one of the [four hundred thousand words in Lia's chart] reflected its author's intelligence, training, and good intentions, but not a single one dealt with the Lees' perception of their daughter's illness.[10]

Today, because health and illness are increasingly defined and treated within certain cultural contexts, more physicians realize that a patient's cultural background must be included in their assessment. Many Western-trained physicians sneer at traditional healing systems, believing that Western biomedicine is far superior. However, Arthur Kleinman, M.D., a medical anthropologist, conducted a study comparing Taiwanese patients treated by Western medicine and those treated by traditional methods. He found that, statistically, the number of people cured by each were within a few percentage points of each other. Follow-up studies confirmed his findings.[11]

Our understanding of epilepsy is still evolving. It does seem that cultural attitudes toward a particular illness impact the ways in which people are treated for that illness—indeed, whether it's considered an illness at all. Much of this book is about incorporating treatments of other, older cultures, whose attitudes and treatments for epilepsy often reflect a deeper understanding of our physical and spiritual needs.

CHAPTER 3

Understanding the Nature of Epilepsy

You can even be angry at your disability, but you would have no reason to be angry at yourself. You didn't cause it.
—ROBERT FRIED, PH.D.

Although having epilepsy can certainly have a negative effect on psychological well-being, epilepsy is not a form of mental illness. Nor is epilepsy a disease. Rather, it is a disorder of the central nervous system that causes recurring seizures. The word *epilepsy* derives from the ancient Greek word *epilepsia*, meaning "to be seized by forces from without." But these forces are very much within us. Epilepsy, also called a seizure disorder, is defined as a chronic condition that produces sudden disturbances in the normal electrical function of the brain, which can cause muscle spasms, confusion, sudden falls, uncontrolled body movements, or loss of consciousness.

The Brain: Gateway to the Body

In ancient Greece, prior to the discovery of the true functions of the brain, the heart was considered to be the seat of reason. Today, neuroscientists know that the brain and spinal cord comprise the central nervous system. Researchers have learned that the brain is made up of several "command centers" that have diverse, though equally important, functions in human survival. Following is a basic description of the fundamental subdivisions of the brain.

The Structure of the Brain

Our brains are composed of approximately 60 percent fat. However, this isn't the same kind of fat found in the abdomen, thighs, or buttocks. From what researchers have discovered, this is structural fat that forms three-dimensional cell membranes and governs nerve-cell function.

The brain is made up of three major components: the brain stem, the cerebellum, and the cerebrum. The spinal cord is attached to the brain by the brain stem, which regulates vital body functions that we're not consciously aware of, such as breathing and heartbeat. The brain stem also controls the functions necessary for arousal to keep us awake and alert.

At the back of the head, located behind the brain stem, is the cerebellum. This structure controls balance and muscular coordination. The cerebellum integrates information from the muscles, joints, and tendons to help the body produce accurate movements. Once the cerebellum "learns" a physical activity, it is able to store that knowledge and recall the information every time that particular activity is performed.

The cerebrum is the part of the brain involved with intelligence. This is the largest segment of the brain, accounting for about

85 percent of the brain's total weight. The cerebrum is divided into two hemispheres, the right and the left. These divisions are joined by the corpus callosum, a bundle of nerve fibers that allows information to be transferred between the two sides of the brain. The outer covering of the cerebrum is composed of a layer of densely packed and interconnected cells called the cerebral cortex, commonly referred to as our "gray matter." Researchers believe that long-term memory is stored in the cortex.

Neuroscientists have identified four lobes within the cerebral hemispheres, each with specific functions:

- Temporal lobe: controls memories, sexual feelings, hearing, smells, and tastes
- Frontal lobe: controls personality, emotions, and movement
- Parietal lobe: receives and interprets sensory information, such as touch, pain, and body temperature
- Occipital lobe: coordinates visual activity

A seizure may affect part or all of the brain. Depending on which part of the brain is affected, a person having a seizure may experience different kinds of sensations. For example, someone whose seizures begin in the temporal lobe might experience an unusual smell.

There's evidence that seizures may have an impact on the hippocampus. Located beneath the cerebrum, the hippocampus is involved in learning and memory storage. It acts as a kind of holding site for working memory before the information is either stored permanently as long-term memory in the cerebral cortex or cleared away to make room for new information. In one study of thirty-five people with uncontrolled complex partial seizures originating in the temporal lobe of the brain, researchers found that the hippocampus was significantly smaller in epileptics compared to nonepileptics.[1]

Neurons: The Basic Units of Brain Function

Brain researchers estimate that human beings are born with 100 billion brain cells, or neurons. Individual neurons are the basic unit of nervous-system functions. Until recently, scientists believed that the number of neurons we're born with was the same as what we died with, give or take a few billion. However, recent discoveries have disclosed that the brain can generate new cells, especially in the cortex and hippocampus. Research has also shown that the brain has hundreds of thousands—possibly millions—of stem cells that can differentiate into fully mature neurons long after birth, even into adulthood. These are especially numerous in the hippocampus.

We lose nearly one hundred thousand neurons every day—more if our brain is subjected to environmental toxins, alcohol, hard drugs, stress, or nutritional deficiencies. However, even at such a rate of loss, it's estimated that people have about 96 billion neurons left by the time they reach a hundred years of age.

Researchers are learning more about brain plasticity, the process by which the brain's neural circuits are "wired" and "rewired." While a child's brain grows fastest before about age three, recent research indicates that it continues to grow into adolescence. Brain-scan studies indicate that the amount of gray matter in some areas of the brain can nearly double within a year, followed by a loss of tissue as unneeded cells are purged and the brain continues to organize itself. This may help to explain why many children apparently outgrow their seizures or their seizure patterns change. For instance, in benign childhood epilepsy, also known as Rolandic epilepsy, seizures almost always disappear after adolescence.[2] A number of children no longer experience seizures but have migraine headaches instead.

Scientists are discovering that adults' brains, too, are continually changing, growing, and being rewired. Our brains are highly adaptable throughout our lives. The principal stimuli for such plasticity appear to be through neurotransmitters and electrical activity of the neurons.

A neuron has three components: one main cell body and two branches, one outgoing (the axon) and the other incoming (the dendrite), which serve as communication links with other nerve cells. Each neuron fires, generating small electrical bursts called nerve impulses that move from neuron to neuron to communicate with the body's central nervous system. The axon and dendrite have multiple connector points so that a neuron can receive and send numerous and simultaneous messages, rapidly picking up electrical impulses. While there is an electrical current generated, the impulse is actually a chemical message.

Messages are transmitted in one direction only, from the axon of one neuron to the dendrite of the next neuron. The space where the axon establishes a connection with the dendrite is called the synapse. (A typical human brain has about 100 trillion synapses.) Each neuron is connected to hundreds of other neurons by anywhere from 1,000 to 10,000 synapses that communicate to each other through chemicals called neurotransmitters. So far, scientists have identified about a hundred neurotransmitters. One of the major neurotransmitters is serotonin, which helps regulate sleep and arousal. Researchers believe that we need adequate levels of serotonin to prevent depression. Another, gamma-aminobutyric acid (GABA), is an important inhibitory neurotransmitter.

Neurotransmitters: Chemical Messengers

Trillions of chemical messages are being transmitted through the brain every second. Such messages from neuron to neuron wouldn't be possible without neurotransmitters, which bridge the gap between adjacent neurons. Made from a variety of proteins, such as enzymes and amino acids, neurotransmitters play a crucial role in the functions of the brain and the nervous system as a whole.

Researchers don't fully understand the ways in which an imbalance of neurotransmitters may cause seizures, but they do know that neurotransmitters create two categories of effect: excitation or inhibition. One neurotransmitter, for example, will tell a neuron to fire, or discharge; another one will tell it not to. (It takes approximately one–one thousandth of a second for a neuron to fire.) This complex yet orderly interconnectedness of cells and chemicals enables us to complete a number of tasks simultaneously. For example, when I ride my bicycle, the nerve cells in my occipital lobe (the part of the brain that controls vision) discharge as I focus on stop signs, cars, and other bicycles, while nerve cells in the parts of the brain that control movement tell my legs to move so I can pedal. Meanwhile, neurons that activate speech, hunger, or urination don't discharge. As long as the excitation and inhibition processes are maintained, my body remains balanced on the bike.

Neurotransmitters, it seems, play a vital role in whether or not a seizure occurs. A seizure begins when groups of neurons within the brain become overstimulated. This may occur, for instance, in response to blinking lights, low blood sugar, or a variety of biochemical imbalances. Some people's seizures are triggered by scar tissue caused by high fever, injury, or a brain tumor. As the neurons discharge excessively, excitatory neurotransmitters tell neurons to fire and inhibitory neurotransmitters tell them not to. If the inhibitory neurotransmitters are able to keep the discharges contained to one area of the brain, a person may experience a brief alteration in consciousness, such as an absence seizure or a myoclonic muscle jerk. But if the neurons are firing very rapidly and the discharges spread throughout the brain, a tonic-clonic seizure occurs. This causes a person to lose consciousness. When this happens, the brain undergoes acute biochemical changes. The brain's metabolic rate speeds up and, with this, glucose and oxygen consumption increases. The oxygen delivery system can't keep up with the huge demands being made by the seizing brain, so the brain becomes starved for oxygen (a person's face might turn blue) and must shift its metabolism to a far less efficient energy-producing system called glycosis. As a consequence, lactic acid builds up in the brain and if the seizure is not stopped, as in *status epilepticus*, the neurons begin to die. But for the vast majority of people, a seizure stops on its own. Currently, there is no way to stop a seizure, other than emergency administration of certain drugs, such as valium; once it has begun, it runs its course. The inhibitory neurotransmitters finally quell it, like firefighters dousing a fire.

A seizure is a symptom and not an illness in itself. It indicates that something has gone awry within the brain. There are different types of seizures and a single person may experience more than one type.

Classification of Seizures

Since the nineteenth century, neurologists have created precise diagnostic definitions of seizures and types of epilepsy. The International Classification of Seizures identifies about forty types of epilepsy.

Allan B. Aven, M.D., who has tested many people with epilepsy for allergies, has a different point of view. He writes:

The various types and subtypes of seizure disorders are merely an artificial way of classification. I think we are really dealing in most cases with the same basic disorder, and whether a person has petit mal or grand mal makes no difference as far as my approach goes, because all this represents localized inflammatory reaction of the brain upon exposure to a specific allergen.[3]

Over the past decade, the names of some seizures have changed, creating confusion among doctors and patients alike. For example, petit mal (French for "little illness") seizures are now referred to as absence seizures because they involve a brief loss of consciousness. Grand mal (French for "big illness") seizures are now called tonic-clonic; tonic refers to the stiffening of the body, clonic refers to the jerking of the body.

Seizures are divided into categories based upon the cause. Seizure characteristics and terms can be rather difficult to follow and they may seem to a lay person like hairsplitting, but these differences can play an important role in the treatment of the disorder.

Idiopathic vs. Symptomatic Seizures

To begin with, physicians try to determine the cause of the seizures. In symptomatic, or secondary, epilepsy, the cause of the seizure is known, such as a stroke, tumor, brain lesion, poisoning, infection, or brain trauma. With idiopathic, or primary, epilepsy, there appears to be no definitive cause for the seizures. This leaves some patients very frustrated. As writer Jeff Morgan, who has idiopathic epilepsy, describes it: "The doctors are idiots and the treatment is pathetic." About 70 percent of people with epilepsy fall (no pun intended) into this category.

I find it surprising that the medical establishment has been content to relegate 70 percent of seizures to the idiopathic, or "unknown causes," category. A number of health-care practitioners and researchers have found that hypoglycemia, nutritional deficiencies, food allergies, exposure to pesticides, and other conditions can cause recurrent seizures. I suspect that if the medical establishment didn't limit possible causes to only those conditions measurable by heavy machinery, the percentage of people with idiopathic epilepsy would decrease and the term *idiopathic* would perhaps be redefined.

The Difference Between Partial and Generalized Seizures

Seizures are also categorized according to their origin: partial or generalized. Partial seizures result from an abnormal discharge in one part of the brain, and generalized seizures are caused by abnormal discharges all over the brain.

Partial Seizures

Partial seizures (sometimes called *focal*) are divided into simple partial and complex partial. Simple partial seizures occur when neurons in just one part of the brain discharge and therefore don't cause a person to lose consciousness. Complex partial seizures (formerly called psychomotor seizures) do affect consciousness. Because these discharges occur in parts of the brain that control seeing, hearing, memory, taste, or feeling, a person generally experiences brief changes in the way things look, sound, taste, or feel. As one person said, "Water just doesn't taste the same afterwards."

A simple partial could be, for example, a tickling sensation on your arm, a bright light, a strong scent, or uncontrolled body movements, such as clapping hands or smacking lips. A person may see people or objects that are not there or hear strange sounds or feel as though what is happening has happened before (as in déjà vu). Someone having such a seizure might mistake this seizure activity as a sign of mental illness.

If excited neurons in one part of the brain "recruit" other neurons, without the necessary inhibitory neurons to stop them, a partial seizure can spread all over the brain and progress to a generalized tonic-clonic seizure. When that happens, the simple partial is what is called an *aura* (from the Greek word for wind). An aura is a forewarning of a seizure that will affect more areas of the body. When such a warning occurs, a person can sit or lie down and sometimes even consciously stop the seizure. (For more information on auras and stopping seizures, see Chapter 10.)

Complex partial seizures affect only certain parts of the body, but they do alter consciousness. Usually lasting from one to three seconds, they can cause confusion, loss of awareness, or aimless movements, such as picking at clothes or wandering aimlessly. Sometimes embarrassing behaviors occur during a complex partial, including undressing or urination, which the person does not remember afterward. Complex partials are sometimes mistaken for alcohol or drug intoxication because confusion after a complex partial may last for some time.

Generalized Seizures

Whereas partial seizures begin locally in a specific part of the brain and then spread, generalized seizures don't have an identifiable focal origin. Neurons discharge all over the brain simultaneously and affect the entire body. Absence, tonic-clonic, and myoclonic seizures are the most common generalized seizures.

Absence seizures are blank spells—a loss of awareness, staring, blinking, or slight twitching—that last for a few seconds. A person is temporarily out of contact but doesn't lose consciousness. This type of seizure may occur dozens or even hundreds of times a day, is often hard to recognize, and may be mistaken for daydreaming or inattentiveness, particularly in children.

Tonic-clonic seizures occur when all the neurons in the brain suddenly discharge. This is the type most often associated with epilepsy, although less than 25 percent of all people with epilepsy actually experience such seizures. The tonic (stiffening) phase begins when the person cries out as air rushes out of the lungs. At that point, the person loses consciousness, falls down, and the body becomes rigid. Then the clonic (jerking) phase begins. As muscles twitch and teeth are clenched, breathing becomes irregular and may even stop briefly, mimicking death. The person may bite his or her tongue or lose control of the bladder or bowels. Gradually, the jerking movements slow down and consciousness returns.

During a seizure, there are dramatic changes in blood flow to the brain due to shallow or stopped breathing. If you could see an x-ray of the brain at the beginning of a seizure, it would look like there was no blood flowing there; the brain blanches. Then there's a surge of blood, as blood flow to the brain increases to protect the brain. At this point a person's face may turn blue because the blood vessels in the skin constrict to allow more blood to flow to the brain.

A tonic-clonic seizure usually lasts one to five minutes, and when the person recovers consciousness he or she may be confused, have a headache, or want to sleep. It may take from ten to fifteen minutes for full consciousness to return; confusion and fatigue may persist for hours or days.

There has been general consensus among the medical community that seizures don't injure the brain or result in a decrease in alertness or intelligence. (Although, as stated earlier, researchers studying people with uncontrolled complex partial seizures originating in the temporal lobe found that, on average, the hippocampus was significantly smaller in people who had epilepsy compared with those who didn't.) Seizures are rarely life-threatening. However, if a seizure lasts more than several minutes, or if one seizure follows another, a person is said to be in *status epilepticus*. Because the body doesn't have enough time to recover normal breathing and heart function, a person in *status epilepticus* may die. If you witness this, call an ambulance immediately. (See First Aid for Seizures at the end of this chapter.)

Myoclonic seizures are most common in children and teenagers. These cause brief muscle jerks, called myoclonic jerks, that last from a fraction of a second to a few seconds. Sometimes the brief muscle jerks cause a person to fall. Sometimes, if discharges spread across the brain, a person may also have an absence or tonic-clonic seizure.

Some less-common types of generalized seizures include:

- Infantile spasms: sudden jerking seizures or shaking usually beginning in infants between the ages of four and twelve months
- Atonic epilepsy: loss of muscle tone, causing a person to fall down
- Akinetic epilepsy: loss of movement, causing a person to drop objects
- Cursive epilepsy: frantic running
- Gelastic epilepsy: uncontrollable laughing
- Photosensitive epilepsy: tonic-clonic, absence, or myoclonic seizures occurring in response to flickering or flashing lights or patterns of color; also called reflex epilepsy

Other Considerations

Following are several conditions that often affect people with epilepsy. This is certainly not a complete list, but these are the ones that have been fairly well researched.

Photosensitivity

In December 1997, emergency rooms all over Japan were deluged with nearly seven hundred children who had suffered convulsions, fainting spells, vomiting, blurred vision, or other symptoms while watching the popular television cartoon "Pokémon." During the cartoon, a creature scared off an enemy with his bright, flashing eyes. This incident, recorded in media worldwide, brought attention to photosensitivity, or reflex epilepsy.

It's estimated that 3 to 5 percent of people with epilepsy have photosensitive epilepsy or pattern-sensitive epilepsy. Seizures can be caused by a variety of visual stimuli, such as flickering or flashing lights; sunlight reflected on water, trees, or buildings; unique patterns, such as windshield wipers or escalator steps; or unusual patterns on glass. The longer a person is exposed to these triggers, the greater the chance of inducing a seizure. Even some people who don't have epilepsy are photosensitive, as with the children watching "Pokémon." And certainly, hours of looking at computer monitors causes a great deal of eyestrain and headaches for people in general.

Fast-paced screen changes on television screens, bright screens, and flickering patterns have all been shown to trigger seizures. Television commercials and programs use many of these "light percussive" effects. Robert Grossman, a neurosurgeon at Baylor College of Medicine in Houston, Texas, says that when we look at a television, computer, video game, or the flashing lights of an ambulance, these "flashing lights seem to entrain brain rhythms." He explains that when people are exposed to light flashing at roughly the same frequency as brain waves, the brain's natural rhythms may synchronize to the artificial stimulus. Then each time the light flashes, more and more of the brain starts firing.[4] Brain cells can become overexcited and if the brain's inhibitory system doesn't kick in, a seizure occurs.

Flicker is not perceptible at frequencies of about one hundred flashes per second, but it nevertheless affects the firing of cells in the retina and subcortical structures of the brain. Cathode-ray tubes, used in most television sets and desktop computers, emit a beam of electrons that illuminate phosphors on the inside of the screen as the beam sweeps back and forth. I usually close my eyes each time I click the mouse for screen changes; otherwise, it hurts my eyes.

Interestingly, this type of epilepsy is reportedly higher in children and young people; in addition, studies have shown that one in four people lose their photosensitivity, usually before the age of thirty. This is not always the case, however. For instance, I have photosensitive epilepsy, but it wasn't diagnosed until I was in my late thirties, after I had a seizure from watching flickering candles.

Researchers have evidence that mothers who are photosensitive have a one-in-four chance of having a photosensitive child—and it seems likely that siblings of the mother will also be photosensitive.[5] There's not sufficient evidence on the probability of fathers having photosensitive children.

Negotiating Your Way Around the Lights   The lines that make up the picture on a television screen are refreshed twenty-five times per second, and the whole screen flashes fifty times per second. Both sources of flicker can cause seizures. The rapid imperceptible flicker from visual display terminals and fluorescent lighting affects eye movements. It can be difficult to avoid the flickering lights that surround us daily, but for anyone who is photosensitive, it may be imperative. Jenny Gristock, a researcher at the Science Policy Research Unit at the University of Sussex in England, offers these suggestions to photosensitive adults and children to reduce seizure frequency:

- Watch television in a well-lit room; sit about six to eight feet away from an ordinary TV.
- Consider using a high-frequency (100 Hz) television or one with a smaller screen. (Interestingly, it's rare for seizures to be triggered by films in the cinema.)
- If you are exposed to a light trigger, cover one eye with the palm of your hand. This will prevent half of the neurons from being exposed and getting excited. (Of course, you can always cover both eyes if you don't need to view it.)

Fluorescent Lights   Fluorescent lighting is known to be a significant trigger of seizures for those who are photosensitive. And it's difficult to avoid, especially since, in offices, stores, and schools, it's used almost exclusively. Incandescent lighting comes from a small filament inside the lightbulb and has little flicker, whereas fluorescent lights pulse end-to-end, flashing 120 times per second. Our eyes may not perceive 120 flashes per second, but our brains do. If you are photosensitive, you should limit your exposure to fluorescent lighting. If you have an office or cubicle at work, consider using an incandescent lamp to offset the fluorescent lighting that is usually provided. Place the lamp at forehead level so one light fills your field of vision. Ask to be near a window, too.

Computers   A growing body of evidence shows that prolonged computer use causes visual stress and creates undesirable visual adaptations, including nearsightedness. The sense of sight is a fragile system. It's hard to avoid using computers, especially for work, and so many people, including nonepileptic computer users, have injuries stemming from consistent use of the equipment. For example, since computers have become popular, carpal tunnel syndrome, caused by making repetitive strokes, has become common. And a study conducted by the Kaiser Permanente medical program in California found that women using video display terminals (VDTs) for more than twenty hours a week during the first trimester of pregnancy were twice as likely to miscarry as those not using them or using them less frequently.[6]

We are expected to accommodate ourselves to the equipment when the equipment should be accommodated to us. Computers and office furniture are becoming more ergonomic, but we still have a long way to go. Here are a few suggestions from Jenny Gristock to help you make computer use more comfortable:

- Make sure you are in a well-lit room.
- Adjust the computer's refresh rate (the rate at which the screen flashes per minute). A refresh rate of more than 60 Hz is less likely to provoke seizures in most people, although different people are sensitive to different frequencies of flashes. Try 70, 80, and 90 Hz to find out what is most comfortable for you.
- Reduce the brightness of the screen. Monitors with white backgrounds have the most flicker. A screen with a black background with amber, green, or white lettering is best.
- Changing geometric patterns on the screen can trigger seizures, so be wary of them.
- To avoid reflections, position monitors against a light background, as opposed to a dark corner, and in an area where other monitors will not be in your field of view.
- Use clean, correctly focused screens. A viewing distance of about thirty inches for a fourteen-inch monitor is recommended.
- Avoid software and websites that use large, bright display areas or flashing screens. (White-screen word processors are a significant problem.)

Palming

One exercise that will help neutralize stress, eyestrain, and headaches brought on by computer use is known as *palming*. You can palm in your chair at a table or desk. First, rub your hands together to warm them. Close your eyes and cover them with cupped hands so that no light gets in. Then rest the heel of your palms on your cheekbones and cross your hands on your forehead. Do not apply any pressure to the eyes themselves and make sure that the eyelids, eyebrows, and fingers are relaxed. Breathe slowly and deeply. Relax, and imagine you are in a beautiful, tranquil setting. The ideal visualization is of a wide-open setting, such as the ocean or the mountains. Your eyes love the warmth and darkness. Do this for one to ten minutes without stopping. Repeat as many times as you like throughout the day.

- Liquid crystal display (LCD) screens have much less flicker than ordinary screens. Until recently, LCD screens have been used only on laptop computers, but they are now available for desktop use.
- Since tiredness can increase the risk of seizures, try not to work on the computer when you are tired, and take frequent screen breaks.

Another option for protecting against seizures is wearing polarized sunglasses. Polarized sunglasses provide some protection against flickers; ordinary sunglasses don't. Specially prescribed computer eyeglasses have been shown to increase the comfort of VDT users for tracking, fixation, focus change, and peripheral vision. Also, one study indicated that blue sunglasses helped suppress wavelengths that caused seizures.[7]

Now that schools routinely use computers, children who are photosensitive should follow these guidelines and any other recommendations from their physician.

Migraines

An estimated 23 million Americans suffer from migraines. Migraine headaches are characterized by throbbing pain on one or both sides of the head caused by constricted blood vessels. This pain is often accompanied by nausea, vomiting, and an increased sensitivity to light. Migraines may last anywhere from a few hours to several days and can be as disabling as seizures.

A strong relationship between epilepsy and migraines has long been suspected. When I mentioned to Dr. Robert Fried that my mother and sister suffered from migraines, he told me that, if placed on a continuum, epilepsy would be on one end and migraines on the other. I've spoken with several people with epilepsy who told me their mothers suffered from migraines, so there may be a genetic factor.

The largest study ever done on the two disorders found a higher incidence of migraines in people with epilepsy as compared with nonepileptics. Conducted at Columbia University's School of Public Health and the Albert Einstein College of Medicine, the study evaluated 1,947 adults with various types of epilepsy as well as 1,423 of their relatives. Based on the results, the researchers estimate that more than 20 percent of the people with epilepsy had migraines, compared to 11 percent of the general population. Yet only 44 percent of those with both disorders reported ever having been diagnosed with migraines. Because epilepsy is viewed as a more serious disorder, researchers say, physicians often overlook migraines.[8]

Here are some of the other associations between epilepsy and migraines:

- Migraines and seizures can be triggered by food allergies and sensitivities, especially to foods such as sugar, chocolate, dairy, caffeine, and white flour.
- Both can be triggered by sensitivity to bright light.
- Chinese medicine views epilepsy, migraines, and strokes as resulting from pent-up energy from the liver.
- Some drugs, such as phenobarbital and valproate (Depakote), have been used to treat migraines and epilepsy.
- Magnesium deficiency appears to play a role in seizures and migraines. Alexander Mauskop, M.D., director of the New York Headache Center in New York City, says that researchers have found deficiencies of ionized magnesium in 30 to 40 percent of patients with migraines.
- For some women, migraines and/or seizures are affected by their menstrual cycle.
- Some children outgrow their seizures and instead have migraine headaches.
- Migraines and epilepsy can cause visions and hallucinations. For example, Fydor Dostoyefsky had ecstatic religious visions before his seizures, and Hildegard of Bingen, an abbess during the Middle Ages who wrote plays and composed music, was a mystic whose visions are thought to have been triggered by migraine headaches.

In addition, several studies have shown that people with epilepsy tend to have more headaches than people in general. There may be several reasons for this, including the amount of stress involved in having a chronic condition like epilepsy; the use of anti-convulsants, which can cause headaches, especially if the dose is too high; and the fact that headaches frequently follow seizures. Further research into the connections among headaches, migraines, and seizures is definitely needed.

SUDEP

Sudden unexplained death in epilepsy (SUDEP) is thought to account for 5 to 15 percent of the deaths of people with epilepsy. It's been defined as sudden, unexpected, nontraumatic, nondrowning deaths. In addition, research autopsies reveal no anatomical or toxicological cause of death. In one study, 74 percent of deaths ascribed to SUDEP occurred at home, many of the people having died in their sleep. Few of these deaths are witnessed, making it harder to ascribe a cause.

SUDEP risk factors include:

- Early onset of epilepsy
- High number and frequency of seizures
- Polytherapy (taking more than one anticonvulsant at a time)
- Frequent dose changes

Many studies have found men to be more at risk for SUDEP, but in one Swedish study of nearly seven thousand people with epilepsy who had died, researchers found that the rate of SUDEP was similar in men and women. Although taking more than one anticonvulsant simultaneously was found to be a risk factor, researchers reported no increase in SUDEP risk associated with drugs such as phenytoin (Dilantin), carbamazepine (Tegretol), or valproate (Depakote) when used as monotherapy.[9]

While SUDEP is something we should be aware of, we must also know that the studies done so far have not taken into account nutritional, environmental, or lifestyle factors. The underlying causes are still unclear. Such findings also underscore the need to live as full and as healthy a life as possible.

Shame and Depression

The greatest source of shame, say many psychotherapists, is loss of physical control. In Western culture, where bodily control is deemed essential, seizures, especially tonic-clonic, are very frightening. A doctor once told me that people who have physical disabilities often have a deep fear of the supernatural. I have no doubt that this is true—I'm terrified of ghosts—but certainly nonepileptics also fear the supernatural and the unknown. Perhaps our seizures manifest human fears of physical bodies doing what they cannot explain. This might be why people with epilepsy are more often abused and shunned than treated with compassion.

Having or witnessing a seizure makes a lasting impression on our minds, consciously and unconsciously. For the witness, it is like watching a person die, then revive herself—all on her own. (This perspective is probably why some cultures consider those who have seizures as possessing special powers.) For the person who has seizures, the shame and disappointment of somehow being betrayed by our bodies are accompanied by a feeling that we've survived a little death. (One survey of people with epilepsy found that 60 percent expected to die during a seizure.) Curiously, the risk of premature death in people with epilepsy is reportedly two to four times greater than in the general population, particularly among children and young adults. Accidents, brain tumors, respiratory and heart problems, and suicide account for much of this early death.

Epilepsy has been called a "hidden" disorder because most of the time we look no different from anyone else. Yet we're often treated differently in school and at work. Researchers have documented that many people with epilepsy suffer from depression. One study, discussed in "Depression in Epilepsy" by M. F. Mendez, compared epileptics with paraplegics and found that depression was almost twice as prevalent among the epileptic individuals. Suicide attempts were four times as frequent.[10] Are we depressed because we have epilepsy? Or do we have seizures because we are depressed? What roles do medications, family interactions, and lowered expectations play? These are questions that are yet unanswered.

Barbara Young, M.Ed., L.P.C., a counselor in Portland, Oregon, believes that depression and learning disabilities are greater in people with epilepsy. "I believe that such depression is strictly physiological," she says. "Whatever is produced by having seizures produces the depression and perhaps anxiety. Some doctors are beginning to understand that to treat someone with epilepsy, they have to inquire about anxiety and depression. I think it's part of the epilepsy and not a side psychiatric symptom."[11]

A Dutch study comparing the health status of patients with epilepsy with the general population found that people with epilepsy reported less active sports engagement, more fatigue and dizziness, nervousness, sleep disturbance, and excitability. The researchers also found that people with epilepsy showed problems regarding self-confidence and had more psychosocial problems.[12]

Herbalist Susun Weed has commented on what she refers to as "the scientific tradition," which is an obsession with eliminating what is considered bad or undesirable instead of accommodating it: illness is the enemy; club it to death. Although epilepsy has supposedly emerged from the shadows of superstition into the light of modern medicine, it still inspires anger and dread: *anti*epileptic drugs, *anti*epilepsy organizations, the fight *against* epilepsy. For those of us who have seizures, such an attitude contributes to self-hatred and shame, to feeling that our bodies are defective and ugly, and that they betray us. How can we achieve optimal health if we think of health as a fight against our bodies?

First Aid for Seizures

Most people are frightened by seeing someone have an epileptic seizure, but witnesses can do a tremendous service by staying with the person and remaining calm. Afterward, the sufferer will most likely be dazed and confused. Witnesses should remain with the person and reassure that person that he or she is all right. Witnesses should also make sure the epileptic person doesn't wander into a road or near heavy machinery. There is no danger of any onlookers being hurt.

During the seizure

- Try to keep track of the length of the seizure.
- If the person is lying down, turn the person on his or her side.
- Put something soft, like a jacket, under his or her head.
- Clear the person's immediate area of any sharp objects.
- If the person is wearing eyeglasses, remove the glasses.
- Loosen tight clothing.
- Never put anything in the mouth of a person having a seizure. Doing so might result in broken teeth. It's a myth that a person having a seizure is in danger of swallowing his or her tongue.
- Do not try to restrain the person. A seizure must run its course.

After the seizure

- Do not offer any food or drink unless the person is fully awake.
- Allow the person to rest.

Call 911 or an ambulance if

■ The person has seizures lasting more than five minutes
without regaining consciousness.

■ The person is injured, pregnant, has trouble breathing, or
has diabetes.

■ The person requests an ambulance.

Certainly, Western medicine's recognition of epilepsy as a biological disorder has helped us in numerous ways. But conventional
medicine's treating epilepsy merely as a brain malfunction and relying solely on synthetic chemicals to suppress seizures are being ques-
tioned. As our understanding of the brain evolves and as research in
alternative medicine accelerates, more and more people with epilepsy
are changing their views.

Research regarding brain structure and chemistry, seizure triggers, treatment, nutrition, and how epilepsy affects us emotionally
and physically has given us a broader understanding of epilepsy. Such
research, combined with our own personal observations, continues
to provide an array of discoveries, giving us more treatment options.
A growing number of us aren't looking to control our seizures simply by taming our neurons; we want to heal our bodies. The following chapters describe alternative ways—some ancient, some new—to
prevent and treat seizures, enabling us to blend conventional and
alternative therapies to create optimal health.

CHAPTER 4

The Usual Route
Diagnosis and Treatment

You accept the prescription and fill it because the spells are nightmares to you. But your job is just starting. You have to live with your nervous system all the rest of your life.
—LENDON SMITH, M.D., AUTHOR OF *Feed Your Body Right*

If you or anyone you know has a seizure, it's imperative to see a physician, who will give you a thorough physical examination including simple muscle tests to determine whether there's been any motor damage. The physician, usually a neurologist, will also conduct some tests to rule out infections, tumors, and brain damage, and if there is a diagnosis of epilepsy, the tests will help determine which type of epileptic seizure you had.

While most of this book deals with options besides pharmaceuticals, medications do alleviate or eliminate seizures for 50 to 70 percent of people with epilepsy, depending on seizure type, and it is important to know their benefits, as well as their possible side effects. This chapter explains what to expect from a visit to a neurologist, how to prepare for it, the kinds of tests you're likely to undergo, different kinds of medications for particular seizure types, and the side effects of those medications.

Preparing for Your First Visit

Before you go to the doctor, it's important to compile your family medical history as thoroughly as possible. Write down illnesses of family members (for example, a grandmother had Alzheimer's disease, an uncle was a chronic alcoholic). Also write down your own medical history: childhood illnesses, any accidents or surgery, head injuries or birth trauma, and food allergies. Physicians rarely get to see a patient's seizures, so it is helpful for them to have as much information as possible. Keep a notebook handy and write down any information you can about your seizures, such as when they have taken place, if there is any pattern to their occurring, or any eyewitness accounts. Such information will help your doctor determine if you have epilepsy or if there are any other possible causes for your seizures. (Possible causes for seizures include diabetes, alcoholism, and other conditions.)

It may be helpful to bring a friend or spouse with you to the doctor's office. Whenever possible, it's best if both parents accompany a child. Even if the child lives mainly with one parent, it not only calms a child to have both parents nearby, but it also helps to have both parents learn how to deal with seizures. They can ask questions firsthand. Being grounded in the facts enables each parent to teach appropriate first aid for seizures to other family members, babysitters, teachers, and anyone who may regularly be in contact with the child.

If you do have epilepsy, the doctor will make a diagnosis and typically you will return every few months for a checkup. This will help the physician see how you are doing when taking medication, clear up problems you may be experiencing with your prescriptions, and discuss any general problems you may be having. The physician may also want to do an electroencephalogram (EEG) in the office or schedule one to be done at the hospital and will probably give you a prescription for a blood test to check that you don't have too much or too little medication in your bloodstream.

Going to the doctor can be embarrassing, time-consuming, and at times, a burden we don't want to bear. But we can view these visits as learning opportunities. Following are some steps you can take that will make your doctor visits more productive and less painful:

- Never lie to your doctor. If, for example, you lose urine or feces when you have tonic-clonic seizures, say so. Lies have a way of adding up and coming back to haunt you. You may be grossed out by the sordid details of your seizures, but doctors have seen just about everything. (They dissect cadavers in medical schools, remember?) The physician is there to help you, not judge you.
- Never discontinue or lower medication on your own. Always discuss changes in your dosage with your physician first.
- Never hesitate to get a second opinion regarding diagnosis or lab tests or to look for another doctor if you feel uncomfortable with your current one. Most insurance plans will cover second opinions and repeat tests.
- Never be intimidated by your physician or any health-care providers. Their objective should be to provide you with information to help you make choices, not to frighten, upset, or insult you. You shouldn't be leaving a doctor's office more upset than when you entered. If that's happening, look for another physician.

Testing for Epilepsy

Generally, epilepsy is diagnosed by neurologists. They use a variety of brain scans to determine if a person has epilepsy and if so, what type. They rely heavily on the EEG and to a lesser extent on more sophisticated tests. Following are descriptions of these tests:

Electroencephalogram (EEG)

Developed in the 1920s, the EEG is to neurological disorders what the electrocardiogram (EKG) is to the diagnosis of heart problems. During an EEG, electrodes are pasted to strategic spots on the scalp to detect brain-wave patterns that may indicate certain types of epilepsy. A printout of your brain waves indicates whether you have epileptic patterns.

Studies have shown that about 20 percent of people with epilepsy actually have normal EEGs, and so EEG interpretation and diagnosis seem to be something of an art. In particular, the EEG is very sensitive to bodily movements, such as blinking or lip smacking, and such movements can produce false irregularities, which are called artifacts.

Not all EEGs are equal. An EEG requires the placement of twenty-one standard electrodes over the scalp, but these electrodes are not always placed the same. "Although there are general guides," writes Ilo Leppik, M.D., "many laboratories have developed their own specific configurations."[1] Also, while it does pick up the small-voltage activity on the surface of the brain, the EEG does not measure the electrical activity deep within the brain. Hans Berger, who invented the EEG, thought the EEG tracked blood vessels within the brain.

Depending on the results of your EEG, your doctor may refer you for one or more brain scans that will search for structural damage within the brain, such as scars or tumors, which could be causing seizures.

Computerized Tomography (CT or CAT)

This type of brain scan takes x-rays of the brain. The patient lies on a metal cylinder for about twenty minutes while several tiny beams of radiation pass through the brain from various angles. This results in a cross-section of pictures in slices. This unique perspective allows doctors to see all parts of your brain. The pictures are then analyzed by a computer and may show brain injury or abnormalities that otherwise would go undetected.

Magnetic Resonance Imaging (MRI)

Equipped with large magnets and radio waves that take pictures of the brain in great detail, MRIs have even better resolution than CT scans. They're able to detect tumors, multiple sclerosis, or blood-vessel abnormalities, although fewer than 10 percent of adults with epilepsy have detectable tumors or other abnormalities. All MRI machines make very loud noises, and many people use earplugs during the test.

Positron Emission Tomography (PET)

PET scans measure the metabolic activity of the brain. In this procedure, the patient lies on a table that moves through a cylinder, as with the CT scan. The person is injected with a glucose (sugar) solution that also contains a radioactive solution. The machine feeds rays into a computer that analyzes data and produces a three-dimensional picture of the brain. It detects irregularity in blood flow, nerve-cell activity, and the presence of oxygen. Due to the cost of this machinery, this procedure is currently used more for research than clinical purposes.

Glucose-Tolerance Test

Doctors used to refer to hypoglycemia as a "crank" illness, insisting that true hypoglycemia, or low blood sugar, was very rare. But with our diets containing increasing amounts of white flour, processed foods, and sugars, some researchers believe that hypoglycemia is by far the most important metabolic cause of seizures.[2] It's been estimated that between 50 and 90 percent of people with epilepsy have hypoglycemia. In addition, the majority of people with epilepsy have low blood sugar at the time of a seizure.[3]

Even if your physician doesn't recommend it, ask to take a glucose tolerance test. This basically consists of fasting from the night before, then spending the morning in the lab, having nothing but water and your blood drawn every hour to see how fast your levels of glucose rise and fall. It's probably not the most enjoyable three hours you'll ever spend, but it's worthwhile to determine if you are hypoglycemic.

Medical Treatment Options for Epilepsy

While medication is by far the most common form of treatment for epilepsy, you do have options. Here are the pros and cons of the major treatments available from the medical community.

Medications

Anticonvulsant medications do not address the underlying cause of seizures; they only suppress the symptoms: the seizures. Most aim to prevent seizures by reducing the amount of electrical activity in the brain. (Researchers are attempting to identify genes carrying epilepsy in humans to allow for the development of drugs that target epilepsy genes directly. Many believe that current anticonvulsants have significant side effects because they target general neural circuits instead of specific gene defects.) The use of anticonvulsant medication is based on the type of seizure, as well as the risk of acceptable side effects. Doctors agree that it's always best to take as little medication as is necessary, and monotherapy (taking just one anticonvulsant) is preferred. Here are some of the most common drugs, what they are prescribed for, and their possible side effects. Note that brand names are given in parentheses next to the generic form:

- **Carbamazepine (Tegretol):** This medicine is prescribed for partial seizures (especially complex partial seizures), generalized tonic-clonic, and combinations of these seizure types.

  Possible side effects: gastric distress, drowsiness, dizziness, headaches, blurred vision, rashes, photosensitivity. Of particular concern to women, it may decrease effectiveness of oral contraceptives and may cause birth defects.

- **Felbamate (Felbatol):** This drug is used with partial and generalized seizures.

  Possible side effects: insomnia, weight loss, nausea, decreased appetite, dizziness, fatigue. Most serious of all, a number of cases of anemia and hepatitis have been reported, with a rate of aplastic anemia of 1 in 3,000 to 1 in 5,000.

- **Gabapentin (Neurontin):** A newer drug, this GABA-related amino acid is considered particularly useful for people who are already taking medications for other conditions.

  Possible side effects: mild fatigue and dizziness, diarrhea, muscle weakness, dry mouth, sleep disturbances, slurred speech, decreased alertness, tremor, rash, and nausea. Gabapentin in very large doses apparently has little toxicity.

- **Phenobarbital or phenobarbital sodium:** This is a long-acting barbiturate prescribed for generalized tonic-clonic and simple partial seizures.

  Possible side effects: drowsiness, depression, memory problems, poor motor performance; can provoke irritability and exacerbate existing behavioral problems, especially hyperkinesia; may decrease the effectiveness of oral contraceptives.

- **Phenytoin (Dilantin):** This drug is considered useful in generalized tonic-clonic, complex partial, and simple partial seizures.

  Possible side effects: rashes, hyperplasia (gum overgrowth) in 20 to 50 percent of patients; hepatitis, systemic lupus, bone loss; may decrease effectiveness of oral contraceptives.

- **Primidone (Mysoline):** This is used principally in generalized tonic-clonic, complex partial, and simple partial seizures.

  Possible side effects: sedation is common but often diminishes with continued use.

- **Tiagabine (Gabitril):** Another new drug, this one enhances the activity of GABA (gamma-aminobutyric acid; GABA is a major inhibitory neurotransmitter). It is used in the treatment of partial seizures.

  Possible side effects: sleepiness, dizziness, and difficulty with concentration.

- **Topiramate (Topamax):** This medicine appears to act on the central nervous system in several ways, including activation at GABA receptors.

  Possible side effects: dizziness, sleepiness, speech disorders, kidney stones, depression, mood swings. Alcohol should be avoided when taking Topiramate.

- **Valproate (Depakene and Depakote):** This medication is used for atonic, akinetic, absence, myoclonic, and tonic-clonic seizures in generalized idiopathic epilepsy and Lennox-Gastault syndrome.

  Possible side effects: nausea, vomiting, anorexia, heartburn, hepatitis, gastrointestinal disorders, increased appetite with weight gain. In addition, valproate severely depletes L-carnitine levels in the brain, which can significantly interfere with seizure control.

This is by no means a complete list. For more information about anticonvulsant medications and their side effects, consult your doctor or pharmacist. Before taking the generic form of your prescription, be sure to ask your doctor if it is safe. Occasionally, inactive ingredients in generics will affect the way the drug dissolves in your stomach and, therefore, how thoroughly it is absorbed into your blood. Some people taking generic anticonvulsants have developed seizures because the rate of absorption into the bloodstream was not stable. One pharmacist says he no longer carries generic anticonvulsants because certain customers were having problems controlling seizures with them.

Side Effects Generally, drugs are not tested for their long-term effects. But there is ample evidence that long-term use of phenobarbital and Dilantin, two of the most popular anticonvulsants, adversely affects the central and peripheral nervous systems, bone marrow, the immune system, skin and connective tissue, hormones, and metabolism. As was demonstrated in the list above, a number of medications can cause drowsiness, dizziness, and fatigue. In his book *Epilepsy Handbook: A Guide to Understanding Seizure Disorders*, G. I. Sugarman wrote:

Gastrointestinal disturbances may be observed during the administration of practically all medications. Long-term therapy with phenytoin (Dilantin) produces considerable alteration of thyroid hormonal states, particularly in epileptic children. Over 40 percent of individuals undergoing therapy may have decreased levels of calcium and phosphorus and elevated serum alkaline phosphates. Phenytoin decreases absorption of vitamin D (which can lead to bone loss), vitamin C, folate, and calcium.[4]

Anticonvulsants can also cause deficiencies of vitamin B_6, vitamin E, zinc, folic acid, vitamin K, magnesium, and manganese, which may result in disturbances in bone and muscle formation. Carbamazepine (Tegretol), primidone (Mysoline), and phenytoin (Dilantin) reportedly reduce absorption of folic acid. Women who take anticonvulsants during pregnancy have a higher risk of giving birth to a child with birth defects (see Chapter 14).

Chronic folate deficiency can increase the risk of cancer; in women, this is especially associated with cancer of the cervix and breast. Additionally, somewhat unsettling is the type of "filler" ingredients used in these medications. For example, the time-release agents for Dilantin include lactose, confectioners' sugar, and talc. The Dilantin thirty-milligram-capsule band contains FD&C Red No. 3. The Dilantin ten-milligram-capsule shell also contains FD&C Yellow No. 6. These are tiny amounts, but anyone sensitive to these chemicals could be affected by them. Even more disturbing is that intravenous phenytoin contains a mixture of 40 percent glycol (antifreeze) and sodium hydroxide (Drano).[5]

Jill Stansbury, who teaches botanical medicine at the National College of Naturopathic Medicine in Portland, Oregon, says, "Our bodies have a hard time breaking down pharmaceuticals. They can accumulate, cause toxic side effects, and deplete the body's energy resources." An article in the *New England Journal of Medicine* states: "Anticonvulsant drugs used to treat patients with epilepsy have long-term toxic effects." Sometimes the medicine can be worse than the seizures.

Many people with epilepsy dislike taking anticonvulsants, which are sedatives and depressants that affect mood and energy levels. As one neurologist said, "It ain't chicken soup." To avoid unpleasant side effects, or because they feel more creative or sensuous not taking medication, or because the anticonvulsants affect the concentrations of other medications they are taking, many people "forget" to take prescribed medications regularly or stop taking them altogether. But for medication to be effective, your body needs to be on a stable regimen.

Noncompliance is very common. In his book *Contemporary Diagnosis and Management of the Patient with Epilepsy*, Ilo Leppik, M.D., says:

> Depending on the community, as many as 90 percent of patients attending epilepsy clinics have been found to have levels of anticonvulsants below the therapeutic range . . . Therefore, much of the perceived lack of effectiveness observed by patients and physicians could be caused by patients' lack of proper drug compliance.[6]

If you experience unusual syptoms such as nausea, dizziness, or fatigue after taking anticonvulsants, notify your doctor immediately.

Bone Loss   Our teeth and gums can be affected by anticonvulsants, too. In a study of forty people with epilepsy who had been taking phenytoin (Dilantin) or carbamazepine (Tegretol) for an average of eighteen years, both groups had similar amounts of alveolar (pertaining to the jaw section containing the tooth sockets) bone loss. Overall, those taking Dilantin had more hyperplasia, or gum overgrowth.[7]

Normally, when a tooth makes new gums, the old tissue is dissolved. But Dilantin interferes with the enzyme that produces collagen, so gums often grow and swell, creating pockets under each gum where bacteria gather to feed on bone and ligaments. But what makes this so ominous is that such inflammation can cause aggravated bone loss. If enough bone is lost, the tooth has no foundation, causing it to die and fall out. It's imperative to brush often and diligently to remove bacteria underneath the gum line so it has no opportunity to attack the bone. A dentist, periodontist, or dental hygienist can best demonstrate proper dental hygiene.

Studies have shown that many people taking anticonvulsants have bone loss, due mostly to altered calcium metabolism and the effects of the drug on vitamin D metabolism. This is especially worrisome in children, whose bodies are growing; in women, many of whom are at risk for osteoporosis; and the elderly, who are at risk for fractures.

Since sunlight stimulates the production of vitamin D, adequate exposure to sunlight is important (about a half hour daily), as is exercise, which helps prevent bone loss. A number of studies have suggested that supplementing the diet with vitamin D can improve bone-mineral content, especially for those who are institutionalized and are far less likely to get plenty of exercise and exposure to sunlight. Some research also suggests that rinsing the mouth with a liquid preparation of folic acid may help.

A study of forty-six mentally retarded people taking anticonvulsants showed that "in certain teeth there was a smaller root-to-crown ratio . . . The male patients were more affected than the female." Such unusually short roots did not appear to be directly related to Dilantin levels but to gingival overgrowth caused by

Dilantin. Further study of teeth from patients revealed other abnormalities.[8]

Lastly, Hal Huggins, D.D.S., reports that certain conditions, including epilepsy and multiple sclerosis, have improved or disappeared after mercury amalgams have been removed from patients' teeth. Just as mercury has been shown to be toxic to the brain, mercury amalgams, used often in dental fillings, are believed by a growing number of dentists to also be toxic to our systems.[9] These fillings can be removed and replaced with less toxic materials; however, it should be done by a dentist familiar with the procedure, since removing amalgams without taking special precautions can actually increase brain levels of mercury. In addition, special chelation treatments should be used to rid the brain of mercury.

Vagus Nerve Stimulator (VNS)

The vagus nerve stimulator—a flat, round, battery-powered device about the size of a silver dollar, technically called a *neurocybernetic prosthesis*—has been approved by the Food and Drug Administration for use in adolescent and adult people with epilepsy. The VNS is surgically implanted so that it vibrates against the vagus nerve, located near a person's collar bone. Neurologists typically set it to discharge in bursts of about thirty seconds each, every five minutes, twenty-four hours a day. Though scientists don't fully understand how the VNS works, it appears that stimulation of the vagus nerve may disrupt abnormal electrical activity in the brain that causes seizures. Patients can use a handheld magnet for additional stimulation if they feel a seizure coming on. They can also stop stimulation by holding the magnet directly over the device.

Though the VNS rarely results in total reduction of seizures, it may result in a significant reduction. In a study of 454 people with poorly controlled seizures who had the device implanted, half of the participants had at least a 20 percent reduction in the number of seizures per day. In about a quarter of the participants, frequency decreased by more than 50 percent. About 20 percent of the participants experienced a worsening of seizures.[10]

The most frequent side effects of the VNS include a hoarseness of voice, cough, voice changes, and shortness of breath. Some people have reported swallowing difficulties and pain in the throat, ear, or teeth. The device is so new that long-term side effects haven't been documented. Generally, people continue to take medication in addition to having the stimulator.

Surgery

Surgery can benefit people whose seizures arise from a single area of the brain. In particular, people who do not respond to medication and whose seizures are debilitating may opt for surgery—that is, removing the part of the brain from whence the seizures are originating. In the United States, about 1,500 people undergo such surgery each year, and for many, it is successful. Because the brain is so adaptable—especially in children—one or more parts of the brain may take over major functions performed by the removed part. There are three types of surgeries: the lobectomy, in which the temporal lobes are removed; the corpus callostomy, in which the band of thick, white nerve fibers that join the right and left hemispheres is split; and, the most radical, the hemispherectomy, in which one entire side of the brain is removed. Hemispherectomies are mostly done on children because their brains are still growing and are better able to compensate for the missing half. (The empty space eventually fills with fluid.) Over the past fifteen years, this operation has been performed on approximately eighty children by surgeons at Johns Hopkins Hospital in Baltimore.

A study of fifty-eight people—nearly all children—who had hemispherectomies at Johns Hopkins found that twenty-nine patients (54 percent) became seizure free. Thirteen (24 percent) had less severe, nondebilitating seizures after surgery. Twelve children (22 percent) continued to have severe seizures. Four patients died from the operation.[11]

One child who underwent surgery, Maranda Francisco, was experiencing up to 120 seizures a day by the age of four. She was forgetting how to walk, talk, eat, and learn. Surgeons removed the entire left side of Maranda's brain. She no longer had seizures and her speech returned to normal. Despite initial weakness, she regained nearly full use of her right arm and leg. The right side of her brain took over for the missing left, assuming responsibility for her speech, memory, motor control, and learning.[12] Now in high school, Maranda leads an active teenage life.

Physicians usually turn to brain surgery as a last resort and after a great deal of testing. As with any surgery, the risk to existing brain function must be carefully evaluated against potential benefits. Because of the extreme risks involved, it is advisable that anyone considering brain surgery first exhaust all nutritional and pharmacological treatments.

Preparing for Surgery   The body tends to view surgery as an assault, and understandably so. To help surgery patients heal faster, many alternative-health practitioners advocate giving patients extra doses of vitamins, especially magnesium, the B vitamins, and vitamin C, which plays a special role in the brain by controlling glutamate levels and regulating dopamine metabolism.

Judith J. Petry, M.D., medical director of the Vermont Healing Tools Project in Brattleboro, Vermont, consulted medical studies to develop supplement suggestions for people facing surgery. She advises that patients take vitamin C (1,000–2,000 mg daily) before and after surgery to stimulate the immune system. Stick to this dosage until the patient has returned to normal eating habits. She also recommends 25,000 IU of vitamin A daily before and after surgery to help healing and to strengthen the immune system. (At this high dosage, a doctor's supervision is strongly recommended; pregnant women should avoid taking vitamin A altogether.) Dr. Petry also has found that bromelain (500 mg four times a day on an empty stomach) helps reduce inflammation. Patients should begin taking bromelain right after surgery and stop when the swelling has gone down. She warns against taking anything before surgery that thins the blood; this includes vitamin E, garlic, and eicosapentaenoic acid (EPA).[13]

Seattle nutritionist Jerri Spalding Fredin read about the importance of vitamin B_6, magnesium, and vitamin C for surgery patients just before her adult daughter underwent brain surgery. "The day after surgery," Fredin said, "her head blew up like a balloon—the kind of edema I had seen so frequently in brain-surgery patients when I interned at the Mayo Clinic. But I knew that vitamin C acts as an excellent diuretic and that taking vitamin B_6 and magnesium would help. The surgeon had merely placed her on limited fluids— one of the worst things he could have done. . . . After taking C, B_6, and magnesium for fourteen hours, she excreted 600 cc of urine and was immediately taken off limited fluids." She adds that there was another young woman in the hospital about the same age as her daughter who had also undergone brain surgery. "She insisted on gorging herself with milk and in no way was interested in supplements. The other woman felt miserable and looked miserable. My daughter was discharged five days before she was, and we thank our lucky stars that we had courage enough to ignore the ignorance of the neurologists."

Dosages can vary, but if a person hasn't taken vitamin C before, it's best to start with 100 mg daily and work up from there to 500 mg or more; if diarrhea results, the dose is too high. Likewise, since magnesium also affects the bowels, it's best to start out with low dosages and gradually increase to the optimal level. Starting out with 50 mg of the major B vitamins in tablet or capsule form is generally considered safe for most people.

"Sometimes," says Fredin, "it is necessary to begin giving vitamins intravenously as malnourished patients, such as people with epilepsy who have been on anticonvulsants for very long, often have problems absorbing the nutrients when first taken orally. But once some of the vitamins are replenished through IVs, people often have no problems afterward."

Consulting with a nutritionist regarding your nutritional needs before and after surgery may be very helpful. In addition, many hospitals now offer courses in mind-body techniques to help prepare patients for surgery. Though nothing is guaranteed, being prepared physically, mentally, and emotionally undoubtedly provides the best setting for a successful surgery.

Looking at the Alternatives

Not all experts see seizures as simply neurological, caused by defective neurons. Says Peter Van Hazerbeke of the Epilepsy Foundation, "There are at least 150 underlying causes of epilepsy."

Metabolic etiology, or the study of the causes of seizures, has been ongoing for decades. One study, in 1940, conducted by the eminent neurologist William Lennox, stated:

Considering all those links between carbon dioxide (CO_2) and epilepsy, namely (1) the influence of carbon dioxide on the EEG, (2) the abnormal values of carbon dioxide in arterial and jugular blood of patients with petit mals and grand mals, and (3) the abnormal variation of carbon dioxide preceding a grand mal seizure in such a way as to indicate a causal relationship, we may conclude that carbon dioxide plays a significant role in the etiology of epileptic convulsions.[14]

Another point to consider is that it's possible EEG scanners are really tracking blood vessels as they contract and expand. There is clinical research evidence to suggest a strong link between epilepsy and involuntary overbreathing, or hyperventilation. Hyperventilation has been shown to lead to EEG dysrhythmia and seizures. Some researchers propose the theory that there is a mechanism through which a person's stress or anxiety leads to hyperventilation, which in turn lowers carbon dioxide levels, triggering seizures.

If patients ask questions about biofeedback or acupuncture, the standard medical doctor will answer, "It's unproved." Ask a question about the effects of diet or vitamins, and physicians—who receive almost no training in nutrition in medical school—often tell patients that vitamins and supplements aren't necessary. "Just eat a balanced diet," they say. But what is a "balanced" diet? And for whom? Each of us has different nutritional needs. And, unfortunately, few physicians recognize food allergies or sensitivities as a possible cause, or factor in, seizures. They are skeptical of anything that isn't proved by the orthodoxy. By comparison, according to the General Accounting Office, Congress's accounting office, only 20 percent of conventional treatments are proved. "In my opinion," writes James Dalen, M.D., "the principal distinguishing characteristics of unconventional and conventional therapies is their source of introduction. American academic medicine has a bias against outsiders."[15]

Other Options for Treating Seizures

Even if a person's seizures are controlled, by whatever means, that doesn't mean that person is healthy. In the six years that I took anticonvulsants, I had just three seizures. But I was constipated, got frequent headaches and colds, had a poor diet, and the drugs masked my problems. Besides unpleasant side effects, anticonvulsants deplete the body of vitamins and put stress on the liver.

For centuries, people with epilepsy and other illnesses have been treated naturally—with acupuncture, herbs, diet, and rituals, for example—but the Western world has just started taking advantage of these methods again. It's as though we've rediscovered the wheel.

Most physicians equate seizure control with good health. To me, good health comes from a desire to strengthen your body; understanding your body's strengths, weaknesses, and proclivities; and eating foods that make your body stronger. Good health also comes from being in control of your health-care decisions. Devising a health-care plan—what you need physically, emotionally, and mentally—helps you find ways to achieve the best overall health possible.

Andrew Weil, M.D., author of *Spontaneous Healing* and *Six Weeks to Optimum Health*, observes in his article in the magazine *Self Healing*: "There is a huge and embarrassing gap between what patients know and what doctors know about alternative approaches, with more patients asking questions their doctors are simply not trained to answer."[16]

For those who feel these same frustrations with conventional medicine, options do exist. An overview of several other methods of healing, many with long-standing reputations for success, follows:

Integrative, or Complementary, Medicine   Integrative, or complementary, medicine is an energy system of medicine and health care that seeks to combine the best of allopathic, or conventional, medicine and alternative medicine. It spans the biases of medical disciplines and cultures by taking a "whole being" approach to the treatment of the patient as well as the physical disorder. Integrative medicine stresses prevention, self-care, and establishing healing partnerships.

Chinese Medicine   Ancient classifications named seizures after the cry of the animals that the sound of the "epileptic cry" resembled. To the Chinese, medicine is a complex system of treatment that has evolved over thousands of years. It uses diet, herbalism, acupuncture, and exercise to treat a wide variety of ailments. The principal concept of traditional Chinese medicine is that disease is caused by an imbalance of the vital force of energy, or *qi* (sometimes spelled *chi*). The practitioner's aim is to detect and treat imbalances in the flow of *qi* so energy can circulate unblocked throughout the body.

Practitioners of traditional Chinese medicine use diagnostic methods that are very different from those of Western doctors. They observe the patient as a whole, taking into consideration mind, body, spirit, and environmental concerns. (When my acupuncturist reads my pulses, she can feel my heart, spleen, liver, stomach, and kidney energy. This is how she determines where to place the needles.) Like many holistic practices, Chinese medicine is highly individual. Recommendations are made for each person's particular set of symptoms rather than a collective treatment for each ailment.

Homeopathy   Homeopathy is based on the principle of "like cures like" (similar to the theory behind vaccination). In other words, homeopathic remedies that produce a set of symptoms (mental, emotional, and physical) of an ailment in a healthy person can cure those symptoms in the sick. Prescriptions are highly individualized. When deciding on a prescription, a homeopath takes into consideration mental, physical, and emotional symptoms and then prepares remedies from extracts of plants, minerals, and animal and human tissues or secretions, which have been diluted. These stimulate the body's own healing mechanisms.

Naturopathy Naturopathic medicine has been practiced for hundreds of years, even before allopathic (conventional) medicine. Practitioners seek to understand the individual needs of a patient and treat the underlying source of illness, applying treatments that work with the body's natural healing mechanisms. This holistic approach to health includes the physical, mental, emotional, and spiritual aspects of a person.

Naturopaths are the only licensed primary health-care providers with extensive training in therapeutic diets and preventive medicine. Students at naturopathic colleges spend two years studying standard medical science; the following two years they focus on a wide range of natural therapies, including clinical nutrition, botanical medicine, clinical psychology, and traditional Chinese medicine. Practitioners often employ homeopathic remedies or other natural modalities. For example, when one young boy who was having seizures came to see Skye Weintraub, N.D., in Eugene, Oregon, she made several changes to his diet and sent him to an acupuncturist for a series of treatments. Eventually his seizures stopped. "I don't take anybody off anticonvulsants until the treatment regimen is in place," she says. "And then, slowly, I wean them and see if the seizures come back. We've lowered dosages, and some people have gone off drugs altogether."

Ayurvedic Medicine   This ancient Indian form of healing relies on herbal remedies, massage, yoga, and meditation. In Ayurvedic medicine, epilepsy is defined as "a pasmara" (*pa* meaning "negation" or "loss of"and *smara*, meaning "recollection" or "consciousness"). The goal of Ayurvedic medicine is to connect the whole body—physical, mental, and spiritual. In the practice of yoga, positions beneficial to the nervous and circulatory system are recommended, and certain factors such as proper hygiene and balanced diet are considered crucial.

People are often interested in alternative medicine, but we've been trained by the media and the medical profession to think of homeopaths, naturopaths, chiropractors, and so on as quacks and charlatans who are somehow less "legitimate" than medical doctors. Indeed, there are a number of medical doctors who call themselves "quackbusters"; they're dedicated to proving that unorthodox medicine is all quackery, instead of researching methods to define their benefits and weaknesses. (Certainly, blind faith in any form of healing is unwise.) Alternative health care attempts to treat the whole person to restore natural balance and activate the body's own healing mechanisms. It is a principle of science that although something has not been proved, it may still be true. For example, although twenty years ago the value of nutritional supplements was not proved, they still had great value.

To get the care our bodies need, we need to trust ourselves more. Medicine is an art as well as a science. Still, beware of miraculous claims. If something seems too good to be true, it probably is. But if a particular treatment helps you, stick with it. Read. Ask questions. If you have access to the Internet—many libraries have computer access to Medline or other health research programs—you can look up medical journal abstracts and complete articles. Ask friends for recommendations of health-care practitioners. Whether it's your first appointment or your hundredth, you should always prepare for a visit to a neurologist or any health-care provider. Write down any questions you may have for your doctor or nurse. You'll probably be seeing them on a regular basis for tests and checkups.

"Tests don't make the diagnosis," says neurologist Mary Anne Guggenheim. "Talking does." She cautions, "Total seizure control for your goal may not always be wise. Sometimes it is better to contend with an occasional mild seizure than to have the constant debilitating side effects of too much medication. To the best of our knowledge, brief seizures do no brain damage." She stresses the need for the patient to share in the decision and for the physician to remember his oath: "First do no harm."

We've absorbed so many fears and myths about epilepsy. And, naturally, when anyone has an illness, we tend to think the worst, which is why facts can be enormously helpful and grounding. Knowledge is important because not only does it help dispel fears, it also helps us make rational, informed decisions about our health and well-being.

PART II

Nutrition

CHAPTER 5

Food Allergies
and Sensitivities

It is probable that a gut in good working order along its entire length, its membranes intact and its motility normal, is essential to the proper working of the brain.

—FROM THE NEWSLETTER OF THE SCHIZOPHRENIA ASSOCIATION OF GREAT BRITAIN

Allopathic, or conventional, medicine has classified about 70 percent of cases of epilepsy as idiopathic (without any identifiable cause). But in making their diagnosis, most physicians fail to test for food or environmental sensitivities and allergies. However, it has become increasingly evident that allergies and sensitivities—usually to common foods—can be responsible for seizures in a number of people.

Food Allergies

There has been little research into the correlation between food allergy and epilepsy; what information exists is mostly anecdotal case studies. Researchers speculate that some epileptic patients may have allergic reactions in the brain that are similar to the swelling, anoxia, and inflammatory chemical reactions seen at other sites of local allergic reactions.[1] The body becomes much more sensitive to abuses, to the point that just the smell of an allergen can bring on an absence seizure. Researchers who have studied seizures and allergies have stated that when no other cause for seizures can be found, the possibility of food allergy should be explored, especially in children.

When a person is exposed to a substance that is perceived by the immune system to be foreign or harmful, the body produces an antibody specifically against that substance. Antibodies, also known as immunoglobulins, are proteins that detect the presence of foreign substances and then initiate the process of neutralizing and eliminating the substances from the body. In doing so, the antibodies trigger a series of reactions. There are different types of such reactions: some are true allergies and some are sensitivities.

An antigen is any biological substance (a toxin, virus, fungus, bacterium, amoeba, or other protein) that the body comes to regard as foreign and dangerous to itself. An antigen induces a state of cellular sensitivity or immune reaction that tries to neutralize, remove, or destroy the antigen by dispatching antibodies (protein molecules) against it.

Says naturopath Skye Weintraub in "Naturopathy: Another Way of Healing" from the *Epilepsy Wellness Newsletter*:

> People may consume large amounts of food to which they then discover they are allergic. They avoid the food for a few months, and any symptoms they had disappear. Then they discover that a very small portion of the food, far less than they previously ate, will start symptoms again. Apparently, when intake of a food is large and regular the body builds whatever immunity it can. When the food is withdrawn, the immune system no longer needs the protection.

But when even a small amount of the food is then reintroduced, symptoms start.

Wheat

Wheat is one of the major allergic offenders in the American diet.
The main allergy-offending component of wheat (along with rye
and, to a lesser extent, oats and barley) is gluten, the protein-carbo-
hydrate combination that enables wheat flour to rise when baking.
A protein substance called gliadin is the prime allergen within the
gluten. According to a report in *The Lancet*, eighteen different medical conditions have been directly linked to gliadin sensitivity,
including epilepsy, autism, and celiac disease (intestinal malabsorption).[2] However, if a person tests for wheat allergens alone, he or she
may miss food allergies to gliadin. The test may read negative for an

The Rice Cure

Tracey Campbell, a journalist who has epilepsy, traced her
seizures to celiac disease.

> When I started seizing, my husband and I were living in Tai-
> wan. We had exit visa problems, so I relied on local herbalists
> for seizure control for probably about six to eight weeks. One
> of the first guys we went to said I should eat rice for a week,
> as seizures were classified a "digestive disorder" under Chi-
> nese medicine. That sounded pretty wacky at the time, and
> we were thrilled to come back to "conventional" medicine in
> the United States, until I blew through the list of anticonvul-
> sant medications in four weeks and had little or no control.
> Now the eat-rice idea sounds like the smartest thing we heard
> in twenty-five years.

allergy to wheat, while the person is actually allergic to wheat gliadin. A specific test for wheat gliadin can be done to determine an allergy.

Celiac disease, which prevents the absorption of certain nutrients, is thought to be caused by an allergy to wheat. One study, done by the Italian Working Group on Celiac Disease and Epilepsy, found that 77 percent of patients with cerebral calcification and epilepsy also had symptoms of celiac disease.[3] Following a gluten-free diet—eliminating wheat, rye, barley, oats, and buckwheat—is advisable. Grains such as rice, kamut, and spelt do not have gluten.

Milk

Dairy milk contains about twenty-five different proteins; of these, five have been consistently linked with food allergies. Researchers who have tested people for allergies found that a small yet significant percentage tested negative for whole milk but positive for specific proteins found in milk.[4]

"I hold milk and milk products to be absolute poison for anyone with any neurological disorder," says Dr. Robert Fried. "Not only is milk not the good source of calcium everybody holds it to be, it actually depletes calcium because the calcium in the milk is used up in the acid-base balance caused by metabolic acidosis from milk consumption. Acidosis [reduced alkalinity of the blood] is a calamity for seizure sufferers because the kidneys can do only about 35 percent of acid-base balance correction, and the lungs do the rest. And that means hyperventilation—just what we taught you with biofeedback not to do.

"In the presence of metabolic acidosis," he adds, "you have to hyperventilate to restore the balance of hydrogen ions in the blood; this is caught up in the pulmonary carbon dioxide expulsion cycle. Hyperventilation, however, causes significant blood-vessel constriction in the body and in the brain, and thus it jeopardizes oxygen delivery to the brain, which is more sensitive to it than the [rest of the] body. That is why it is used in neurological examinations to produce theta EEG seizure patterns—because it can trigger seizures."[5]

In one study reported in the *Journal of Applied Nutrition*, four epileptic children with autism who were receiving anticonvulsants were treated with either a gluten-free and milk-reduced diet or a milk-free and gluten-reduced diet. Three of the four had a reduction in seizure frequency.[6]

Another study, published in the *Journal of Behavioral Medicine*, reported a three-and-a-half-year-old boy with tuberous sclerosis, mental retardation, and uncontrolled seizures who was placed on the Feingold diet (salicylate and food-additive elimination) three separate times. Each time resulted in substantial reductions in seizure frequency. During a twenty-one-week follow-up, seizure frequency remained low despite the phasing out of one drug, and seizures were reportedly eliminated one year later, although hyperactive behavior was unchanged.[7]

Brain Allergies

A "normal" allergy or sensitivity to a specific substance can cause inflammation of the tissues, resulting in swelling and tenderness. When an allergic reaction occurs in the brain, the swelling happens inside the skull. Brain allergies usually act like regular allergies or sensitivities at first: they just make you feel sick. But after a while, you start to crave the food that is causing the problem. Foods most likely to be involved are those that a person craves and eats in large amounts over a long period of time.

Brain allergies can also affect the central nervous system. The causes of these allergies are usually the same as other allergies, including heavy-metal toxins, imbalances in blood sugar, and foods. The main difference is that they specifically affect brain function. A change in behavior and attitude is often an early sign of a reaction. Ordinary foods such as milk, eggs, and wheat can cause some people to act drunk, be confused, even have epileptic seizures. The most common symptoms of brain allergies in children are fatigue, aggression, irritability, tantrums, depression, learning disorders, and the inability to concentrate. In adults, brain allergies tend to manifest as manic-depressive disorders, various phobias, and certain other mental disorders.[8]

In the majority of central nervous system allergies, a copper imbalance is thought to play a key role. High levels of copper are toxic and may be a principal cause of brain allergies—a hair-mineral analysis can identify this imbalance. Excess copper can cause zinc deficiency, which may result in a rise in sodium levels. And a high sodium level is responsible for many of the symptoms associated with brain allergies.

In her book *Allergies and Holistic Healing*, Skye Weintraub writes:

Some people who have problems with foods or environmental toxins don't break out in a rash, they don't get hay fever, with sneezing and coughing. What is probably happening is that it's all contained in the brain. Maybe the brain is swelling, the circuitry is off. I don't even call it a biochemical imbalance; it's just the allergy is there, and since we can't see the symptoms, all we know is the end results. There are some theories that epilepsy may in fact be the brain allergy. It may have started out like a regular food sensitivity or allergy or maybe the child started out with colic and hives and a lot of the medications they use suppress it, so eventually this is where you ended up. The body had no way of venting, so what did it do? It seized. This is one area that hasn't been addressed. But if you're dealing with food and environmental toxins, then what you hope is, if the symptoms of brain allergies go away and the epilepsy is contained in that, you'll see a difference.[9]

William Philpott, M.D., former director of the Institute of Bio-Ecologic Medicine in Oklahoma City, has estimated that about 50 percent of seizures may be related to maladaptive reactions to foods, chemicals, or inhalants. He treated a six-year-old girl who began having absence seizures at the age of two and a half. Taking the phenobarbital her physician prescribed only worsened her condition, and she developed tonic-clonic seizures upon awakening and usually after meals. She became so uncoordinated and sluggish that teachers labeled her retarded.

When her mother brought her to Dr. Philpott, he tested her for food allergies and she reacted to more than half of all foods— some of which caused her to have seizures. Her worst reaction was to corn, one of her favorite foods. He placed her on a diet devoid of foods she was allergic to and also gave her cystine, an amino acid that helps the body to utilize vitamin B_6. Her improvement was immediate: she began talking in sentences, lost her lethargy, and stopped having seizures.[10]

Testing for Food Allergies

Allergy tests are controversial. Not all are accurate. Sometimes the tests result in false positives (they tell you you're allergic to a particular food, but when you eat it, you have no reaction). In addition, while some allergy symptoms occur within a few hours of exposure to an allergen, others can occur up to seventy-two hours afterward; testing is different for delayed versus immediate reactions. It is best to seek the advice of a health professional who understands the importance of nutrition; beware of anyone promising a quick "cure."

Elimination Diets

If you want to test yourself, the elimination diet may be the best way to detect which foods are causing the problems. This involves removing the suspect food from your diet for four or five days and observing if symptoms improve. When the food is eaten again, see if the original symptoms appear. If they do, you know that you are sensitive to that food. It's important to eliminate one food at a time. This is one of the simplest and most economical methods for determing allergies, but it's not always successful because many people have problems with unsuspected foods.

In one study, for four weeks sixty-three children with epilepsy followed an elimination diet consisting of lamb, chicken, potato, rice, banana, apple, cabbage, sprouts, cauliflower, broccoli, cucumber, celery, carrots, parsnips, water, salt, pepper, pure herbs, calcium, and vitamins. All but eighteen of the children improved on the diet. Of the forty-five epileptic children who also had recurrent migraines, abdominal symptoms, or hyperkinetic behavior, twenty-five became seizure-free and an additional eleven had fewer seizures during diet therapy. Headaches, abdominal pains, and hyperkinetic behavior ceased in all patients whose seizures resolved, as well as in some patients who continued to have seizures. Symptoms were provoked by forty-two different foods, and seizures occurred after ingestion of any of thirty-one various foods.[11]

Most children in this study reacted to several foods. Both those with generalized epilepsy and partial epilepsy improved on the diet. In double-blind, placebo-controlled food challenges (reintroduction of food), symptoms recurred in fifteen out of sixteen children (including seizures in eight cases) after ingestion of offending foods, whereas no symptoms were triggered by a placebo.

Children whose seizures are due to food allergies can be identified by the presence of other potentially food-allergic disorders, such as migraines, abdominal symptoms, or hyperactivity. Researchers urge that the possibility of food allergy be investigated in all children with epilepsy and, when indicated, an elimination diet should be tried.

Self-Testing

One way to determine if you might be allergic to a substance is by taking your pulse when you are around the substance or have ingested it. (This is just another way your body "talks" to you.)

Before testing, avoid any form of the food for at least four days but not more than ten days. When omitting many of the basic foods, such as corn, wheat, yeast, eggs, milk, beef, and pork, be aware that many commercially prepared products contain these ingredients. During a period of food avoidance, it is common to have withdrawal symptoms that usually clear by the end of the third day.

Before starting this test, write down all the symptoms experienced, such as stuffy nose, cough, throat clearing, tiredness, headache, seizures, and so on. On the fifth or sixth day of avoidance, set aside time to perform the test. Take and record your pulse (or the pulse of the individual being tested) for one full minute before eating. Place two fingers over the artery just inside the wrist of the opposite hand (don't use your thumb because it has a pulse of its own). Then eat an ordinary serving of one specific food within a five-minute period. Make sure you eat only the test food. Don't add anything to the food, not even salt. If the food needs to be cooked, then use glass or stainless steel pans and utensils. Use only distilled water during cooking.

Following the meal, take and record the pulse for one full minute every fifteen minutes for up to ninety minutes. If the pulse goes above eighty-four beats per minute, or if there is a variation of more than ten beats per minute, this would suggest a food allergy. A pulse increase without symptoms indicates a probable sensitivity. If definite symptoms occur, the test is positive for that particular food. Observe any symptoms that occur over the next half hour. If you don't observe any symptoms, include the test food with the next meal. Watch for delayed symptoms during the night or the next day.

One-third of allergy-prone people will have an increase in pulse rate, while another one-third will experience a decrease, and the other third will experience no change. You can have a reaction to food for as long as three days after eating it.[12]

Other Allergy Tests

More formal tests include the enzyme-linked immunosorbent assay (ELISA), accurate for immediate (IgE) or delayed (IgG4) allergies. There's also the Immuno 1 Bloodprint test for detecting delayed food allergies; this is a variation of the ELISA test. Also used are electrodermal tests, a technique derived from acupuncture but with no needles used. Instead, an electronic instrument with a handheld electrode applies a weak direct current to the body. It's possible to test most substances with an electrodermal machine, including foods, chemicals, vitamins, medications, and heavy metals. If you want to take one of these tests, speak to your doctor (preferably one who is nutritionally oriented) or a naturopath.

Food Sensitivities

Sensitivities are similar to allergies. Both are bodily reactions to environmental agents such as pollen, mold, dust, and food. A sensitivity is a condition that may come and go with environmental changes, but allergies may be more permanent conditions. The foods you are allergic to should be totally avoided. An allergic condition implies that an altered protein (an antibody) forms either in the blood or in the tissues of the allergic person. A sensitivity does not imply the formation of an antigen-specific antibody but may result from some other circumstance. Many types of sensitivity may not show positive on immunologic tests because these reactions are associated with digestive problems or a toxicity reaction.

The majority of people who have reactions to foods have food sensitivities, not allergies. It is possible to have several major food sensitivities that are causing symptoms. Since there may be no evidence of the allergic reaction in many people with food sensitivities, doctors often conclude that they are suffering from an emotional disorder. Oftentimes such a conclusion is the result of doctors not knowing what to look for or what tests to perform, so instead of treating the food sensitivities, they prescribe drugs.

More and more evidence shows that food sensitivities occur when the digestive system does not function properly. Most people are unaware of the association of foods with reactions because of the delayed symptoms, which may not appear for several hours or several days. Common symptoms include chronic fatigue, arthritis, hives, migraine headaches, asthma, stomach pain, sinus congestion, irritability, hyperactivity, and cerebral allergies. Adverse responses to foods can deeply disturb various delicate biochemical balances in the body.

Any food can cause a reaction but some foods are more likely to cause problems than others. Eating the same food too often is usually what causes sensitivities. In the United States, the most common allergens are dairy, beef, wheat, corn, eggs, chocolate, peanuts, and sugar (these are often present in processed foods, making them hard to avoid). An allergic reaction, as a symptom rather than a disease, may be a sign of a deeper, underlying problem.

Food sensitivities usually disappear with the elimination of the reactive foods from the diet, along with improved dietary habits. These foods can often be reintroduced without recurrence of symptoms by the process of rotating foods in the diet—eating them just every four or five days—and properly cooking and combining foods. This is the best way to prevent food sensitivities from developing in the first place.

While more physicians have now linked food allergies to seizures, Chris M. Reading, M.D., has gone a step further. He has suggested that some of the same hereditary food allergies that cause illness in one member of the family may cause other illnesses in other family members. He proposes that in families with allergy-linked conditions, including epilepsy and alcoholism, it may be more practical to test and treat the entire family.[13]

Dr. Reading believes that deficiencies of vitamins B_1, B_3, B_6, B_{12}, folic acid, and the minerals calcium and magnesium can cause abnormal EEGs or seizures, and that those deficiencies are not necessarily caused by a poor diet. Such deficiencies can also be caused by malabsorption—a damaged intestinal tract unable to properly absorb nutrients after eating foods to which the body is sensitized, such as wheat, corn, or sugar, for example.

Dr. Reading's extensive research of hereditary food allergies and their relation to a number of illnesses resulted in a surprising link between systemic lupus erythematosus (SLE, or lupus), which he believes is caused by food allergy, and epilepsy. "Epilepsy can precede SLE by many years, says Dr. Reading. "Epilepsy can be the first sign of SLE."[14]

The research so far on preventing seizures with a rotation diet and megavitamin therapy is promising and needs to be further explored. Of course, not all seizures are due to allergies or sensitivities. However, while a particular food might not actually be triggering seizures, an allergy or sensitivity may be lowering the seizure threshold. Since the foods people are the most sensitive to are usually their favorite foods and the foods that are most easily obtained, it is difficult to eliminate them from their diets. But alternatives do exist, and the rewards of improved health and fewer seizures are worth the effort. (See Resources for publications that offer ways to change your diet.)

CHAPTER 6

Foods That Harm

In epileptic persons, a change in blood sugar can induce a seizure.

—WILLIAM PHILPOTT, M.D., FROM *Nutrition Guide for
the Prevention and Cure of Common Ailments and Diseases*
BY CARLTON FREDERICKS

According to H. Morrow Brown, M.D., recent research has confirmed that food caused seizures in three-quarters of a large group of epileptic children studied.[1] One boy almost stopped having seizures completely when he was switched to an anticonvulsant containing no azo dyes. The children in the study were suffering from migraines, misbehavior, and epilepsy. The study linked all three problems with food, showing how illnesses of the nervous system can be alleviated by avoiding certain foods or chemicals.

Alcohol

Some scientists believe that many of the symptoms we call alcoholism are the result of an allergy to alcohol, B-complex vitamins, and sugars. Human brain function depends on sugar absorption and utilization and, according to Devi Nambudripad, N.D., a naturopath, sugar digestion and assimilation depend on certain enzymes made from B-complex vitamins. When people have an allergy to B complex and sugar, they may have the tendency to become addicted to alcohol, since alcohol temporarily satisfies the brain's partial need for sugar. (Is it merely a coincidence that alcoholic beverages are made from the grains—such as wheat, corn, and barley—that people are most often allergic to?) A study of chronic alcoholics found that those who had partial seizures often had abnormalities in their EEG, lesions found in CT scans, and previous head injuries.[2]

Alcohol consumption can cause recurring seizures in people not diagnosed with epilepsy. Like sugar, alcohol is absorbed very quickly into the bloodstream. Research conducted by Jean Poulos and Donald Stoddard has shown a correlation between alcohol addiction and blood-sugar problems.[3] They discovered that all of the alcoholics in their research were either hypoglycemic, prediabetic, or diabetic. Another study concluded that sugar, white flour, and refined carbohydrates—staples of the modern American diet—are addictive substances that have similar effects on brain neurotransmitters as alcohol. Sugar and refined carbohydrates increase brain production of dopamine, serotonin, and norepinephrine—which leads to a "high." Abruptly removing these substances from your diet can result in withdrawal symptoms, such as dizziness and depression.

Walter Alvarez, M.D., believed alcoholism to be one of the symptoms of "nonconvulsive" epilepsy. In *Help Your Doctor Help You* he wrote, "While I worked in the gastroenterology section of the Mayo Clinic many nonconvulsive epileptics came to me, usually because of an abdominal discomfort, but never because of convulsions." He found that patients with abdominal discomfort often had abnormal brainwaves and that by prescribing Dilantin he was frequently able to relieve their abdominal pain. In a book on nonconvulsive epilepsy, he wrote:

In 1945, when I abstracted ninety-nine histories of relatives of epileptics, I found that in 38 percent of the families there had been alcoholics. Later, I read L. Marchand's splendid book (*Heredite et Epilepsies*, Paris, 1938) and found how surprised he was to note that a number of epileptologists had found alcoholism in a high percentage of relatives of epileptics—almost half or more than half of the cases. Marchand and others were much impressed by the fact that in many epileptic families there were more alcoholics than epileptics.[4]

Nutritionist Jerri Spalding Fredin, who has petit mal epilepsy and whose younger daughter has epilepsy, speculated on the link between alcoholism and epilepsy in her article "New Hope for People with Epilepsy":

While I knew of no epilepsy on either side of my family, I had traced alcoholism in blood relatives of my ancestors back to post–Revolutionary War days, when Dr. Benjamin Rush made the first national study on alcoholism. My husband also had alcoholism in his family, but he found no epilepsy. . . . After reading what Dr. Alvarez wrote . . . and because there was alcoholism in my family but no epilepsy (before mine) I began to wonder if our daughter's seizures could have been related to some hereditary factor connected with alcohol addiction.[5]

She adds that when she began having nocturnal seizures, she contacted her physician:

Having heard that people with epilepsy should not drink alcohol, I asked him if he thought that the small glass of wine I had been drinking once a day for years might be triggering my seizures. He said alcohol could "lower the seizure threshold"; so I stopped drinking wine—and my seizures stopped.

Kathleen DesMaisons, author of *Potatoes Not Prozac*, theorizes that some people inherit a genetic inability to properly metabolize glucose. Their bodies respond dramatically to the consumption of sugar, releasing beta-endorphins that create cravings for more sugar or alcohol. Actress and model Margaux Hemingway seemed to be a prominent example of the genetic link between alcoholism and epilepsy. One of the few celebrities to publicly discuss her epilepsy, Hemingway wrestled with alcoholism and depression. Her grandfather, the novelist and short-story writer Ernest Hemingway, also suffered from alcoholism and depression. He committed suicide in 1961 at the age of sixty-two. Tragically, in 1999 when she was just forty-one, Margaux also committed suicide; toxicological tests determined her cause of death was an intentional overdose of phenobarbital.

The association of epilepsy with alcoholism has been long and unnecessarily overlooked, and it certainly needs more research. Researchers may well find documentation linking abnormal glucose metabolism not only to seizures but also to the depression experienced by patients with seizures.

Just as coffee drinking is a social ritual, gatherings are often centered around alcohol, and it can be a challenge to go without. I haven't had a drink in fifteen years, and I sometimes wish I could indulge in the occasional beer or glass of wine. But I still attend the parties. I usually bring sparkling water or club soda, and thoughtful hosts will have a bottle of sparkling apple or cranberry cider on hand (looks like a wine spritzer). I don't feel so much like I stand out when I remind myself that lots of people who don't have epilepsy forgo alcohol for health reasons.

Caffeine

It's been estimated that Americans consume over 400 million cups of coffee every day. In most major cities there's a coffee shop on nearly every corner. Like sugar, caffeine is present in many foods, including coffee, chocolate, teas, cola and other soft drinks, headache remedies, and some medications.

Because it is a stimulant, caffeine is best avoided, especially if you have epilepsy. Caffeine may cause damage to neurotransmitters, so that the chemical messages relayed from cell to cell may be slowed or relayed improperly. Overconsumption of caffeine can constrict blood vessels, which means less blood—and oxygen—getting to the brain. Also, just as blood sugar rises when we eat simple carbohydrates, it also rises when we consume caffeine, and that can lead to hypoglycemia.

Caffeine can contribute to many physical and physiological problems, including vitamin and mineral loss, ulcers, sleep disorders, anxiety, and depression.[6] Check food labels to determine if caffeine is an ingredient. You can substitute herbal teas for coffee (though some herbal teas contain caffeine) or try a grain-based coffee substitute, such as Pero or Roma (just make sure it's not a grain you're allergic to!). Ann Louise Gittelman, author of *Super Nutrition for Men*, suggests taking 500 mg of choline three times a day to help ease the caffeine withdrawal. She says that acetylcholine is made from acetyl coenzyme A and choline B, a B vitamin found in high-protein foods such as fish, liver, eggs, soybeans, and peanuts.

Dr. Bernard Green, author of *Getting Over Getting High*, suggests that 2,000 mg of vitamin B_{12} taken in time-release form will provide an energy boost and the mental acuity of a morning cup of coffee. He advises that this be taken with a high-potency B vitamin tablet or a multivitamin and mineral supplement that contains all of the B vitamins.

Too many of us eat a rushed breakfast after too little sleep, grabbing a cup of coffee and perhaps a bagel or pastry on our way to work. A well-digested, nutritious breakfast, such as fresh fruit with cooked cereal (oatmeal or millet, for example), ensures that blood sugar will remain constant throughout the morning and lessens the desire for a quick pick-me-up.

In essence, substances such as caffeine, alcohol, and sugar are neurotoxins. Many health-care practitioners believe that our cravings for them are actually brought on by nutritional deficiencies. We try to counter these deficiencies by taking more of the substance we crave, which provides temporary relief, but in the long run, vital nutrients are depleted, resulting in more craving. Supplying the body with the nutrients it needs is extremely important in getting over addictions and bringing the body back into balance. If the body always has what it needs, it is less likely to create a dependency in the first place.

Sugar

Even though our culture recognizes that sugar is harmful, sweet foods are the easiest, cheapest foods to obtain. From infancy, most of us are hooked on sugar. Studies have shown that excessive amounts can contribute to the development of various health problems, including tooth decay, diabetes, hypoglycemia, and seizures. Yet most of us crave sugar. Sweet foods, like cookies and candy bars, are used as rewards and as comfort foods.

White refined sugar, or sucrose, is present in many canned and processed foods, so sometimes we don't even know we're eating it. So much sugar is added to canned and frozen fruits and vegetables, frozen foods, cereals, and soft drinks that we eat almost as much sugar in these foods as we do in cake and candy. (The next time you reach for a Coca-Cola, remember that you're about to drink the sugar equivalent of a piece of chocolate cake—including the frosting.) It's even in iodized salt; vinegar is used in the processing so sugar is added to remove the bitter taste. It's also used to coat medication tablets, including some anticonvulsants.

White refined sugar provides no vitamins, minerals, enzymes, or fibers that the body needs. It's an antinutrient that uses up the body's vitamin stores, distorts lipid (fats) metabolism, and, importantly, has been implicated in seizures. In 1898, Charles S. Bond, M.D., described a patient, a nine-year-old boy, who developed seizures after eating a great deal of candy and crackers. Dr. Bond wrote that he was "thoroughly convinced that the cortical explosions are induced by the toxic influence of fermenting food in the alimentary canal."[7] Food that ferments, or rots, can cause too much acid in the stomach, leading to gas, indigestion, and stress on the gastrointestinal tract.

In 1910, a physician writing in another medical journal stated, "I have had two cases in which it was clear that a too exclusive or an exaggerated diet of sugary and starchy foods was a cause of epilepsy." The boy "lived practically on 'cakes,' a little breakfast food, etc., with enormous quantities of sugar, syrups, etc. Recovery followed a diet list that excludes the sweets and most of the starches."[8]

Reports such as these surfaced more than one hundred years ago. "Only" forty-two years elapsed between Dr. James Lind's research on the correlation between scurvy and the lack of vitamin C and the British Navy issuing lime juice to its sailors. Why has it taken so long for the American medical profession to accept sugar as a powerful trigger of seizures?

Sugar is also one of the most common allergens. Sugar and sugar substitutes overwork the pancreas, spleen, and liver, lowering resistance to infection. Nutritionist Gary Null says that three ounces of sugar—the amount found in the average candy bar—can suppress immune activity for twenty-four hours. So sugar isn't healthful. But it gets more complicated. When we eat simple carbohydrates (pastries, french fries, pizza) the sugar from these foods gets absorbed too rapidly into the bloodstream and could possibly cause low blood sugar. A steady diet of simple carbohydrates can cause constipation. Both low blood sugar and constipation are factors in seizures.

Not All Carbohydrates Are Created Equal

All parts of the body—organs, tissues, and muscles—must have a steady supply of energy so they can function. Unlike other parts of the body, which can also use fats and amino acids for energy, the central nervous system depends almost exclusively on glucose, a simple sugar. Since the brain is "command central," it's perhaps not surprising that it uses more energy than any other organ in the body. Trillions of chemical messages are being transmitted throughout the brain every second. While accounting for only about 2 percent of our body weight, our brains use about 20 percent of all oxygen and 25 percent of all glucose.[9]

Carbohydrates are broken down in the intestines into simple sugars. Eventually, all these sugars are converted into the simplest sugar, glucose, in the liver. Glucose, the main sugar used for fuel, circulates throughout the body through the bloodstream. The series of reactions needed to break down glucose in the brain also depends on an adequate supply of vitamins, minerals, and trace elements. For the body to function properly, there must always be a certain amount of glucose in the bloodstream. When that level drops below what is needed, it can result in low blood sugar, or hypoglycemia, which, as was stated earlier, has been indicated as a possible cause of seizures.

Complex carbohydrates, found in most fruits, vegetables, and whole grains, break down into glucose more slowly than other carbohydrates. This ensures that the body, and particularly the brain, has a steady supply of glucose. An important aspect of complex carbohydrates is that most are high in fiber. Fiber, essentially, is the part of the carbohydrates that our bodies can't digest. Yet foods high in fiber are of tremendous value. They "scrub" the walls of the colon and bowel, fill us up, and are absorbed at an even, consistent rate, ensuring a stable supply of energy through glucose. Most people need about 20 to 30 g of fiber a day.

Complex whole foods, including fruits, vegetables, and grains that are fresh, baked, or stir-fried, supply fiber. But in processed foods (canned, dried, or precooked) the fiber has already been broken down, so the sugar content is absorbed into our blood much more rapidly, temporarily raising the level of glucose instead of supplying the constant flow that the body really needs. Therefore, it is advisable to stay away from processed foods, particularly if you are hypoglycemic, epileptic, or both.

The Importance of Fiber

Constipation has been shown to be a factor in seizures. It is notable that some anticonvulsants can cause constipation, and it is a common problem in children with epilepsy. Eating enough fiber will facilitate bowel movements, which is important because the longer the stool stays in the intestines, the more likely unwanted waste will be absorbed back into the blood, where it will travel to the brain.

Our livers process nutrients and detoxify our blood. But as Betty Kamen, Ph.D., has written, when the liver is overwhelmed with toxins, it becomes more difficult to remove toxins. Any toxic substances that escape the liver ultimately go to the brain, which is far more sensitive to toxins than any other organ. The blood-brain barrier filters out toxins in the bloodstream; however, many toxins can penetrate this barrier. Having regular bowel movements helps cleanse the body, and eating enough fiber will help in avoiding constipation. Eating whole grains, fruits, vegetables, bran (wheat, oat, or rice), oat germ, and wheat germ should help with irregularity, as will prune juice and psyllium seeds. If you continue to have problems with constipation after increasing your fiber intake, you might try taking a lemon enema before going to bed—combine the juice of two lemons (lemon helps the body cleanse itself) and two quarts of water and follow the directions on the box containing the enema pouch.

Hypoglycemia

Some researchers believe that hypoglycemia is by far the most important metabolic cause of seizures. Dr. Lendon Smith states in his book *Feed Your Body Right* that hypoglycemia has been known to be a factor in seizures since 1934.[10] For example, according to R. B. Allen in his article "Nutrition Aspects of Epilepsy," 50 to 90 percent of people with epilepsy have constant or periodic low blood sugar. And 70 percent or more of people with epilepsy have abnormal glucose tolerance tests.[11] Perhaps most notable, glucose levels are unusually low in most people just before they have a seizure.

Hypoglycemia is, very simply, a deficiency of glucose in the blood. While all foods contain energy, different foods affect blood sugar (the amount of glucose in the blood) in different ways. Simple sugars such as soft drinks and refined white flour are absorbed from the intestines into the bloodstream very quickly. When traditional diets were based on complex carbohydrates, hypoglycemia was little known. But in our modern way of eating, a steady diet of processed foods and sweets can cause the body to overreact and produce much more insulin than the body actually needs. The blood is flooded with insulin. This results in a large amount of blood sugar being absorbed quickly, resulting in a high. When the blood sugar drops quickly, the entire body is thrown off kilter. Blood sugar can fall so low that the brain doesn't get its needed fuel, causing depression, anxiety, fatigue, shakiness, headache, inability to concentrate, and even seizures.

Although the correlation between blood-sugar abnormalities and epilepsy seems well documented, the actual mechanism hasn't yet been determined. It's been suggested that low blood sugar could impair production of adenosine triphosphate (ATP), a compound generated by the metabolism of food. All cells in the body use ATP for energy. Low blood sugar reduces the efficacy of the ATP sodium pump, and this defective sodium pump allows increased intracellular sodium concentrations, which depolarize the cell membrane, thus lowering the firing threshold.[12]

In a healthy person, as blood glucose rises after a meal, the pancreas gradually releases insulin to regulate glucose levels. When a person has hypoglycemia, the pancreas overresponds to carbohydrates and creates first an elevation, then a sharp drop, in blood sugar.

Hypoglycemia is usually determined by glucose-tolerance tests. These are relatively simple fasting tests in which a person is given 100 g of glucose to drink. Then, blood glucose and insulin are measured every hour for five to six hours. A nonhypoglycemic will maintain relatively constant blood-sugar levels. But someone with hypoglycemia will have rapid drops in blood sugar. Home glucose-monitoring kits, which allow people to gauge the amount of glucose in their blood, are now available at most drugstores.

In her article "New Hope for People with Epilepsy," nutritionist Jerri Spalding Fredin writes: "From books I learned that some seizure victims no longer had seizures after being treated for hypoglycemia, and that the brain waves of those with hypoglycemia were similar to those of persons afflicted with petit mal/absence seizures."[13]

It is important to remember that hypoglycemia is reversible. Many people who have hypoglycemia have improved when their diets were high in complex carbohydrates. Russell Blaylock, M.D., says, "I have seen quite a few patients suffering from hypoglycemia in my practice. All improved dramatically when placed on diets high in complex carbohydrates and low in simple sugars." Standard diets for hypoglycemia spread the day's food intake over three meals and three snacks. Brad Wallum, M.D., an endocrinologist with Overlake Hospital in Bellevue, Washington, says he aims at about 45 percent of calories from complex carbohydrates, including whole-grain bread, potatoes, rice, and vegetables, 25 percent from protein, and 30 percent from fats. "The trick is to spread them over six or more meals and balance carbohydrates with enough protein and fats to slow the digestive process," says Wallum. He compares this meal plan to a diabetic diet.

A Sweet Is a Sweet Is a Sweet

There are plenty of sugar substitutes available. When baking, I use fruit juice in place of sugar. Canning fruits usually requires sugar, but my friend Sharon uses frozen juice concentrate (apple, white grape, or pear). She mixes a twelve-ounce container with a gallon of water, heats it following particular canning directions, and uses it as syrup. Pam Krause, author of *Pam's Favorite Recipes*, has devised a 50/50 sweetener that is two and a half cups raisins and two and a half cups apple juice, mixed in the blender. Nutritionist Gary Null suggests using fruit juices made from soaked dried fruits to sweeten dishes. Since dried fruits are high in natural sugars, a little will go a long way.

But sugar is still sugar. All sweeteners affect blood sugar (except stevia). Don't fall into the trap of substituting "natural" sugars for sucrose. Watch out for simple or concentrated sugars and keep sugar to a minimum. Once you cut down or eliminate the amount of sugar you eat, you'll notice how overly sweet many foods taste. Following is a list of common and uncommon sweeteners, some of which have nutritional value.

- **Sucrose,** or white table sugar, comes from sugarcane and sugar beets but is devoid of the vitamins and minerals found in the whole plant. Such refined sugar tends to strain the body's digestive system.
- **Saccharin** is an artificial sweetener. Packets of Sweet 'n' Low, which contains saccharin, carry a warning that it has been implicated as a cause of cancer.
- **Corn syrups** are highly allergenic and addictive for many people. They're found in many products, including aspirin, bacon, baking mixes, beer, breads, processed meats, and canned peas; the glue on envelopes, stamps, and stickers may contain corn syrup.
- **Sorbitol** is another artificial sweetener. It is absorbed more slowly than sugar, but the caloric value is the same if it escapes breakdown in the liver. Nutritionist Carlton Fredericks believed it could wreak havoc with the eyes and contribute directly to cataract formation.
- **Fructose** is the type of sugar found in fruits. Naturally occurring fructose accounts for only about 5 percent of net weight in most fruits. Commercial fructose is refined sugar usually made from corn. High-fructose corn syrup, which is added to many processed foods, has been identified as a causative factor in heart disease.
- **Honey** is a natural sweetener refined by bees. It is 40 percent naturally occurring fructose and contains B-complex vitamins and vitamins C, D, and E. It is about twice as sweet as sugar, which deters many people from consuming it in large amounts. Unfiltered, unheated, and unprocessed honey is most nutritious, with its enzymes and vitamins still intact. Because of the natural bacteria that live in honey, it should never be given to babies under one year of age.
- **Barley malt syrup** is made from sprouted barley and contains potassium. Brown rice syrup is made from ground brown rice

that is mixed with enzymes. If you are grain sensitive, look for brands that are gluten free and have not been mixed with wheat, oats, barley, or rye. Rice and barley malt syrups have the consistency of thick honey and work well in sauces and pastries.

- **Carob, or St. John's Bread,** is a powder that comes from the dried pods of the carob tree. It tastes a lot like chocolate but it has no caffeine and contains protein, B vitamins, calcium, magnesium, and potassium. One cup of carob powder contains 2 g of fat, compared to 108 g of fat in cocoa. Carob powder, flour, and candy are available in health-food stores.
- **Stevia** is a natural sweetener that has been classified by the Food and Drug Administration (FDA) as a food additive rather than a food. This means that it can be sold as a dietary supplement but cannot be included as an ingredient in food products. It can be purchased at health-food stores or can be grown at home. Scientific research has indicated that stevia may help regulate blood sugar because it isn't digested by the body. Stevia is calorie free and tends to reduce cravings for sweets and fatty foods. It also contains proteins, fiber, iron, calcium, and other nutrients. It tastes thirty times sweeter than sugar and is now approved for use as an ingredient in more than seventy Japanese food products, including candy, ice cream, yogurt, and pickles. Ground stevia can be sprinkled over vegetables, cereals, and salads.
- **Maple syrup** is very sweet and should be used sparingly. It reportedly contains the trace mineral zinc.
- **Blackstrap molasses** contains iron, calcium, and B vitamins.
- **Sorghum syrup** is made from juice extracted from sorghum cane. It contains potassium, calcium, and iron.
- **Granulated cane sugar** (Sucanat) has a lower sucrose level than refined sugars and contains molasses. It also contains trace elements.

Excitotoxins

There's a class of chemicals used as food additives that neuroscientists have dubbed *excitotoxins*, so named because they overstimulate neurons in the brain. This poses a distinct danger, especially to people with epilepsy. The most common excitotoxins are glutamate, found in monosodium glutamate (MSG), and aspartate, found in aspartame products such as NutraSweet and Equal. According to Dr. Russell Blaylock, author of *Excitotoxins: The Taste That Kills*, when brain cells are exposed to these substances, they can become overly excited and fire very rapidly until they are exhausted to death. Not only are brain cells lost, but other cells within the brain are damaged.

Since glutamate and aspartate are two of the most common excitatory neurotransmitters, our brains normally contain high concentrations of these chemicals. So it may be surprising that glutamate and aspartate could be toxic. But our nervous system maintains an ongoing, delicate balance of positive and negative impulses. When the amount of glutamate and aspartate rises above certain levels, too many neurons get excited and fire. Without inhibitory transmitters to balance their firing, they fire and fire until they are damaged or die.[14]

Normally, these neurotransmitters' positive and negative impulses maintain a balance within the brain, which is also helped by blood-brain barriers in each neuron. These barriers act as gatekeepers, allowing certain substances into the brain's environment and excluding those that are deemed harmful. However, some parts of the brain, such as the hypothalamus (which controls body temperature and many other metabolic processes) have no blood-brain barrier, so they are directly affected by various toxins and excitatory proteins in the blood. When either glutamate or aspartate is allowed to build up outside the neuron, they become toxic.

Our nervous system carefully controls the amounts of glutamate and aspartate in a number of ways, the most important of
which is a kind of pumping system that rapidly removes them from
extracellular space, preventing a buildup. If, for example, glutamate
is not removed, even small elevations in glutamate levels can result
in a state of excitotoxicity. Excitotoxicity also results with mercury
poisoning, excess iron levels in the brain, low magnesium, and low
glucose levels.

Research has shown that even those areas of the brain with an
intact blood-brain barrier can be vulnerable to excitotoxins from
food. When blood levels of glutamate are high, the glutamate can
slowly seep through the barrier and enter the brain. In fact, it has
been shown to accumulate in the brain for as long as twenty-four
hours. In addition, glutamate from the blood can infiltrate the "protected" areas of the brain by entering through sections without a barrier protection, such as the hypothalamus, a so-called back door
entry.

Conditions such as physical stress, head trauma, hypertension,
diabetes, infection, hypoglycemia, seizures, and angina can cause the
barrier to break down and allow substances normally filtered out
by the blood-brain barrier to enter neurons. Disruptions of this
balance can cause symptoms as slight as a tremor, twitch, or absence
seizure or as severe as a tonic-clonic seizure. But consuming foods
containing excitotoxins over time has been shown to have long-
lasting, deleterious effects in some individuals. Researchers have
linked a number of disorders, including migraine headaches, brain
tumors, seizures, developmental brain disorders, and Alzheimer's
disease, to eating foods containing excitotoxins. Excitotoxin injury
to the brain appears to be a common denominator for a multitude
of injuries and disorders of the nervous system and plays a key role
in seizures.

Monosodium Glutamate

Monosodium glutamate, or MSG, is a taste enhancer popularly known as the cause of "Chinese restaurant syndrome," which causes some people to suffer rashes, headaches, dizziness, or seizures after eating food flavored with MSG. But MSG is used in thousands of processed foods, including most salad dressings, snack foods, frozen entrees (especially diet foods), ice cream, frozen yogurt, and low-fat foods. It was even in a chicken pox vaccine! Foods whose labels say "No MSG" sometimes contain large amounts of glutamate. Be wary of anything containing the words *flavoring* or *natural flavoring* in the list of ingredients. Also be wary of the "light" foods with reduced fat because manufacturers usually replace the lost flavor with flavor-enhancing glutamate. MSG may also be listed on labels as "hydrolyzed vegetable protein," "vegetable protein," and "spices." Or it may not be listed at all. Under Food and Drug Administration guidelines, if an ingredient makes up less than 1 percent of a food, it doesn't have to be listed.

High doses of glutamate can cause rapid cell death, whereas low concentrations may not kill the neurons outright but may severely impair their ability to function. In studies in which glutamate was injected directly into the brains of animals, or given orally, it caused seizures in various animal species.

There has been a great deal of controversy surrounding glutamate since it was approved by the Food and Drug Administration in the 1940s. In July 1995, the Life Sciences Research Office of the Federation of American Societies for Experimental Biology prepared what was supposed to be a definitive report for the FDA on the question of the safety of MSG. While the report seemed to say that MSG was safe, it stated that "motor disturbances and changes in seizure threshold have been noted in numerous studies." The report also stated that there were numerous studies confirming the link between changes in brain chemistry and ingestion of MSG. This is of particular concern for children because the documented neurochemical changes involved the neurotransmitters responsible for learning, memory, and behavior control. Many infant feeding formulas, vitamins, and medicines for children contain high levels of glutamate. This is especially worrisome because a child's developing brain is four times more sensitive to excitotoxins than an adult brain.[15] At least one study has shown that feeding MSG to a pregnant animal significantly lowers the infant's seizure threshold. Also, by altering how brain pathways form, glutamate can increase the risk of neurological disorders, including seizures. (Incidentally, Dr. Blaylock points out that all of the newer anticonvulsant medications are glutamate-blocking drugs. Whether these provide any protection from eating MSG is a question left unanswered.)

Aspartame

This artificial sweetener has been accused of causing more than ninety side effects and contributing to brain damage, seizures, and cancer. Aspartame has been shown to increase brain levels of phenylalanine and methanol; methanol is converted within the tissues of the brain into formic acid and formaldehyde, both powerful neurotoxins. According to H. J. Roberts, an aspartame expert and author of *Aspartame NutraSweet: Is It Safe?*, more than 80 percent of food-additive complaints that the FDA has received have been regarding aspartame, complaints ranging from headaches, migraines, and breathing difficulties to seizures and other neurological disorders. Several of Roberts's patients whose seizures were controlled on phenytoin (Dilantin) found that the medication lost its antiseizure effect while they were using aspartame. Roberts says it may render some young children more vulnerable to seizures. He writes of a two-year-old child who suffered seizures within ten minutes of chewing aspartame-sweetened acetaminophen (Tylenol).

Even people who don't have seizure disorders have had seizures after eating foods containing aspartame. More than six hundred commercial airline pilots have reported symptoms, including some reports of tonic-clonic seizures in the cockpit, after eating food containing aspartame.[16]

The NutraSweet company claims that more than two hundred scientific studies have established aspartame's safety. However, NutraSweet funded most of those studies. It's disturbing that the FDA accepted studies conducted by one of the major companies with a huge financial stake in the outcome, tests that many independent scientists found to be seriously flawed. For example, in a number of experiments, it was not disclosed that an unusually high percentage of test animals developed brain tumors and that some died. (Although mice who took aspartame had exceptionally high rates of brain tumors, there is no proof that aspartame causes brain tumors in humans. Yet Dr. Blaylock notes that from 1973 to 1990 brain tumors in people over the age of sixty-five increased 67 percent.) It's also disturbing that some government officials who approved NutraSweet wound up working for NutraSweet and its affiliates, including Monsanto, NutraSweet's parent company.

Even moderate hypoglycemia can magnify the toxicity of excitotoxins. The hypoglycemic state makes the brain even more vulnerable to the effects of excitotoxins. Hypoglycemia can cause neurons to fire spontaneously. It is now known that anything that can make the neuron fire will remove the magnesium blockage of the calcium channel, which regulates the entry of calcium into a cell. Simply having low energy reserves in the cell could cause a neuron to fire spontaneously, which would then relieve the magnesium blockade of the calcium channel. When this occurs, large amounts of calcium pour into the channel, triggering a number of chemical reactions that cause the cell to die. When energy supplies are low, even low doses of glutamate and aspartate can kill neurons because the cell's protective mechanisms require large amounts of energy to work. Research shows it is the hippocampus that can be injured first and most severely, while the cerebellum is spared.[17]

Another reason that using glutamate and aspartate as food additives can be harmful is that they stimulate the production of free radicals. Free radicals are unstable molecules that the entire body creates in minute quantities during metabolism. These free radicals, which produce oxidation reactions, attack and damage cells. High levels of oxygen can be destructive to our bodies, just as fats and oils turn rancid when exposed to the air for very long. Our bodies protect themselves by neutralizing these molecules with other molecules called antioxidants (meaning "anti-oxygen"), which can easily penetrate the blood-brain barrier and enter the neurons that need them. Fortunately, you can increase the levels of these antioxidant nutrients in your brain and whole body by including in your diet foods and supplements rich in vitamins C and E, as well as vitamins A, D, and K, and minerals such as magnesium, zinc, chromium, and selenium. (One study found epileptic patients had significantly lower selenium levels than any other group except those with cancer.[18]) One of the brain's best antioxidant protectors is glutathione. Brain glutathione can be increased by taking the supplements N-acetyl-L-carnitine (NAC) and alpha-lipoic acid.

Magnesium plays a vital role in brain protection and is a major modulator of brain activity. Significant protection of brain cells is seen when magnesium is taken after excitotoxin exposure. Magnesium can significantly protect against seizures and enhances the effectiveness of seizure medications, thereby improving seizure control.

Excitotoxins have a cumulative effect, and their effects are multiplied by the addition of other excitotoxins within one's diet, so chronic exposure to them can cause increasing damage. Experimental evidence shows that glutamate and aspartate affect the neurological development of the brain. Additionally, aspartame is known to make the EEG discharges worse in children with certain types of epilepsy. Excitotoxins penetrate the placenta so pregnant women should assiduously avoid foods containing MSG and NutraSweet. In fact, the placenta can concentrate these toxic proteins in the baby's brain so that the baby's blood levels are actually higher than the mother's.

Avoiding excitotoxins is difficult since they're usually hard to identify in processed or restaurant food. And if we suffer a reaction to a food, we face more confusion about the cause: is it glutamate, aspartate, pesticides, other additives, or the food itself? It has been demonstrated that toxins often have additive effects and that even when taken in individual, subtoxic levels, full toxicity can result if they are combined in a meal. When MSG or aspartame is used with exposure to pesticides, other food toxins, or pollutants, significant damage to the cells of the body can result. MSG has been shown to significantly increase free radical formation in a number of cell types besides neurons. Since glycine, a neurotransmitter, can also be an excitotoxin, people with seizures should be warned against using glycine supplements.

While ingredients remain hidden, the best way to avoid the addition of excitotoxins is to prepare your own food from fresh ingredients. And when you use processed foods, eat only those that you trust are free of toxins. You're more likely to find these in health-food stores than in supermarkets, but don't assume that all products in health-food stores are free of glutamate or aspartame. Glutamate can be found in anything protein fortified, enzyme modified, and fermented.

While all of this sounds alarmist and pessimistic, it is only meant to inform. Our bodies and brains are delicate systems, but they are also incredibly resilient. Unquestionably, much of our food supply contains a multitude of harmful substances. But by refusing to buy these products and by asking questions in food co-ops, supermarkets, and restaurants, you can help protect your health and the health of your family. In addition, buying organic food and growing more of your own fruits and vegetables will ensure that you know where, and how, the food you eat is grown.

CHAPTER 7

Foods That Heal

Let thy food be thy medicine and thy medicine be thy food.
—HIPPOCRATES, FROM "ON THE SACRED DISEASE"

While anticonvulsants often prevent seizures, the little research that has been done in this area indicates that they often deplete our bodies of essential vitamins and minerals. In this way, whatever problems or deficiencies that might be causing or exacerbating our seizures may in turn be exacerbated by anticonvulsant medications.

This chapter discusses nutrition and the vital role nutrition plays in our health and well-being. Evidence indicates epilepsy and seizure disorders may respond very well to nutritional therapy. Nutritional needs vary from person to person, and improving our overall health can only help prevent seizures.

Epileptic seizures can have many triggers. If an underlying imbalance or weakness is present, a seizure can be triggered by factors such as foods, chemicals, even trauma and emotional excitement. Still, even though reactions to foods can trigger epileptic episodes, your physician might not ask what you eat or what you feed your child. He or she may inquire about your employment or your home life but not how you nourish your body. It's like a car mechanic neglecting to ask how often you change the oil in your car or failing to check the transmission fluid.

Although few physicians in the Western world recognize food as having anything to do with seizures, other cultures have recognized this relationship throughout the centuries. With the discovery of anticonvulsant medications earlier this century, Western medicine turned away from the possibility of food-related seizures. However, many people who suffer from epilepsy think what they eat may have a lot to do with the timing and severity of their seizures.

Are You Meeting Your Nutritional Needs?

We usually know when something is wrong. Our bodies are very smart. It's important to pay attention to their symptoms or signals. How do we know we're getting what we need? It helps to learn about nutrition: read books, go to seminars and lectures, attend health fairs, ask questions. If your health-insurance plan allows, or if you can afford it, you might benefit from seeing a nutritionist or naturopath as well.

While it's always beneficial to eat wholesome food, state of mind can also affect our nutrition. If our minds and bodies are locked in conflict or struggle or unhappiness, it doesn't always allow for the proper digestion and absorption of nutrients. You can have the best diet in the world, but if you are self-abusive, anxious, or unhappy, your nervous system and digestive system may suffer. Also keep in mind that certain vitamins may be helpful for some people but not well absorbed by others.

Nutrients That Raise the Seizure Threshold

Dr. William Philpott found that one-half of the epileptic patients he studied had abnormal carbohydrate metabolism, low B_6, low calcium, and low magnesium, which, says Dr. Lendon Smith, can allow a susceptible person to have seizures.[1] Dr. Smith adds that lead poisoning could make a person even more susceptible, and that low blood sugar will trigger an attack. To determine if you have a lowered seizure threshold, Dr. Smith finds helpful a good laboratory screen test of the blood and a hair analysis, with special interest in the heavy metals and levels of manganese, magnesium, and calcium.

"The nutritional approach," says Dr. Smith, "would be the standard no-sugar, no-junk diet, with six nibbled meals a day." For daily supplementation, he suggests 1,000 mg of calcium; 500 mg of magnesium; B complex with 500 to 1,500 mg or more of B_6, especially if dream recall is poor; 1 to 5 mg of folic acid; 5 to 15 mg of manganese; 200 to 400 mcg of biotin; and 30 mg of zinc. He adds that taurine and glutamic acid have been shown to help reduce seizures.

Vitamins

Vitamins contribute to good health by regulating metabolism and assisting the numerous biochemical processes that release energy from digested food. (All B vitamins are extremely important to the function of a healthy central nervous system.) While drugs operate as blocking agents and can function alone, vitamins act as facilitating or enabling agents and require the presence of other nutrients. Therefore, their effectiveness is limited when other nutrients are in short supply. To make matters more complicated, anticonvulsant medication tends to interfere with the body's absorption of a number of vitamins and minerals, including vitamin D, calcium, and folic acid, so supplementation can improve overall body health and seizure control. If you commit to a program of supplementary nutrients, preferably under direction of a nutritionist or physician, you will need to maintain this regimen for several weeks or months to assess its effectiveness. Following is information about a number of vitamins that have been shown to be of particular benefit in preventing seizures.

Vitamin B_6 (Pyridoxine)

A lack of B_6 and magnesium has been closely associated with convulsions, which may be prevented by an adequate supply of these nutrients. In addition, taking anticonvulsants can deplete your body of B_6 and folate (another B vitamin).

According to naturopath Gaetano Morello, there are two known types of vitamin B_6–related seizures in newborns and infants under eighteen months of age: B_6-deficient and B_6-dependent. They have similar neurological symptoms, EEG abnormalities, and a prognosis of mental retardation if not treated.

The diagnosis of pyridoxine dependency, says Dr. Morello, should be suspected in every infant with convulsions in the first eighteen months of life. Certain clinical features may be indicative, including:

- Seizures of unknown origin in a previously normal infant without an abnormal gestational or perinatal history
- A history of severe convulsive disorders, in both the family and the individual
- The occurrence of long-lasting focal or unilateral seizures, often with partial preservation of consciousness

- Irritability, restlessness, crying, and vomiting preceding the actual seizure[2]

Since medical literature lists atypical presentations of pyridoxine-responsive seizures, researchers have recommended that an empirical trial of pyridoxine be conducted on any newborn or infant with long-lasting convulsions, especially when no clear etiology, or cause, is present. A 100 to 200 mg intravenous dose of pyridoxine or 20 mg dose every five minutes to a total of 200 mg is often recommended. If the seizures stop, it is likely that the child has pyridoxine-responsive seizures.[3] The chance to identify a pyridoxine-responsive seizure is lost if pyridoxine is given with, or after, most anticonvulsant drugs.

While B_6-deficient seizures can be stopped with the administration of dietary amounts of pyridoxine, B_6-dependent seizures reportedly require continuous high-dose supplementation in the range of 25 to 50 mg per day.[4]

Although the mechanism by which B_6 decreases seizure activity is not fully understood, researchers believe it is related to its role as a necessary cofactor in the metabolism of a variety of neurotransmitters, including gamma-aminobutyric acid (GABA), an important inhibitory neurotransmitter. It's been suggested that for some people whose brain chemistry results in reduced GABA, higher levels of B_6 are required. B_6 needs adequate magnesium in order to be properly absorbed.

One uncontrolled study (that is, no controls, or people without epilepsy, were included) of infants and children with infantile spasms found improvement in two to fourteen days using oral pyridoxine phosphate (20 to 50 mg/kg). Three participants had complete relief, six showed transient relief, and eight showed marked reduction in seizures and improvement in their EEGs. However, some adverse reactions, such as nausea and vomiting, were seen.[5]

Nutritionist Jerri Spalding Fredin thinks that most Americans—not just people with epilepsy—are deficient in folic acid and vitamin B_6, which, she supposes, accounts for the high percentage of heart disease in the United States compared with countries where there is a higher intake of fresh vegetables (good sources of B vitamins) and a lower intake of animal proteins (which require a higher intake of B vitamins to control the blood homocysteine level).

Joe Graedon and Teresa Graedon, Ph.D., authors of *Deadly Drug Interactions: The People's Pharmacy Guide*, write:

> Taking Dilantin can deplete your body of vitamin B_6 and folate (another B vitamin). Talk to your doctor about finding the proper amount of B_6 and folate to take. If you are megadosing with more than 80 mg a day of B_6 or 2 mg daily of folate, Dilantin could be only half as effective and seizures may occur. (Note that these levels are much higher than the federal government's recommended Daily Values of 2 mg for vitamin B_6 and 400 mcg for folate.) Finding out what is enough or too much is a little bit like walking a tightrope.[6]

While promising results have been obtained by the administration of vitamin B_6, B_6 administration to those with epilepsy must be strictly monitored and it's best to seek the care of a nutritionally trained professional. When large doses of B_6 are given, the other B vitamins should accompany it, especially B_2 and pantothenic acid. If a person's health doesn't improve, poor absorption may be the reason.

Niacin (Vitamin B_3)

Supplementation may bolster the effect of anticonvulsants. Abram Hoffer, M.D., researcher and author of many books on nutrition and medicine, as well as a founding father of the alternative-health movement, clinically observed several patients who were unable to achieve control with anticonvulsants because the required dosages made them so drowsy and sluggish that they were unable to function normally. They were given 1 g of niacin three times daily. After they had taken the niacin for several months, the dosages of anticonvulsants could be slowly reduced, while the patients were monitored carefully for an increase in seizure frequency.[7]

Choline

The B vitamin choline has exhibited some anticonvulsant activity in human and animal studies. It aids in building and maintaining a healthy nervous system and works to remove fat from individual cells and the liver. Authors of one study found that choline may be beneficial in treating complex partial seizures. They advise starting with 4 g daily. Increase to between 12 and 16 g daily by the third month.[8]

Vitamin C

Vitamin C strengthens the immune system. It's important to proper functioning of the adrenal gland (the "antistress" gland) and therefore also helps combat stress, a leading cause of seizures. In addition, vitamin C plays a special role in the brain by controlling glutamate levels, thereby helping to prevent damage by excitotoxins. The recommended daily allowance for vitamin C is 45 mg, but many nutritionists believe much higher doses are necessary and advise those with epilepsy to take 2,000 to 7,000 mg daily, in separate doses.

Folic Acid (Folate)

A deficiency of folic acid appears to play a role in seizure activity, but there is conflicting information. While people taking the folate-depleting anticonvulsants often are deficient in folic acid and should take folic acid supplements, for some people, folic acid supplementation causes an increase in seizures. Thus, discussing possible folic acid supplements with a qualified health practitioner may guide your decision to take the supplement. According to Margaret Watkins, an epidemiologist with the Center for Disease Control's Birth Defects and Developmental Disabilities Division, "Folate is the form naturally occurring in food; folic acid is the synthetic version." This slight difference may play a role in why supplementation does not work for everyone.

According to several researchers, people who are currently taking anticonvulsant medication may be at increased risk for cardiovascular disease from elevated homocysteine due to lowered folate levels in their blood. Homocysteine is an amino acid by-product of protein breakdown. In one study evaluating plasma total homocysteine and serum folate levels in more than a hundred epileptic patients taking anticonvulsant medications, a significant inverse correlation was found between folate and total homocysteine levels. The difference was more pronounced in the group of older people.

All the folic acid–deficient patients had received multiple anticonvulsants for more than seven years. Folic supplementation at 10 to 20 mg a day reduced homocysteine levels and increased folic acid to the normal range. Folic acid and homocysteine should be evaluated in epileptic patients to help prevent thrombosis due to hyperhomocysteinemia, or elevated homocysteine levels. Patients with elevated homocysteine due to lowered folate levels should consider supplementing their diets with folic acid to reduce their risk for cardiovascular disease.

Cooked lentils, garbanzo beans, spinach, and green peas are foods with the highest amount of folate. Supplementation of 0.5 mg folic acid is recommended for people with epilepsy unless otherwise advised.

Vitamin D

The association of anticonvulsant drugs with disorders of mineral metabolism, including hypocalcemia and rickets, is well documented. Conflicting results have been published concerning the serum levels of vitamin D in patients with epilepsy. Studies have reported increased, normal, and decreased levels. Anticonvulsant drugs interfere with vitamin D and calcium metabolism in some manner not well understood.[9]

Adequate exposure to sunlight is important (about a half hour daily) because it supplies our bodies with vitamin D. Supplemental vitamin D intake is recommended when climatic conditions or a person's lifestyle does not allow adequate exposure to sunlight. In one study, supplementing the diet of twenty-three people with epilepsy with 4,000 to 16,000 IU of vitamin D resulted in a significant decrease in the number of seizures, indicating a possible therapeutic effect.[10] Such high doses, however, can be toxic and require careful monitoring.

Vitamin E

Vitamin E and selenium function synergistically in many ways. Vitamin E deficiency is known to produce seizures, and a number of studies have shown people with epilepsy to be low in vitamin E and selenium. Supplementation with vitamin E and selenium may result in fewer seizures.

In an experimental study, discussed in "Is There a Role for Vitamin E Therapy in Epilepsy?" by A. Ogunmekan, eighteen children between the ages of five and twelve who had at least six tonic-clonic seizures per month were given 400 mg of vitamin E a day in addition to their medication. After two months, sixteen had improved seizure control, with a 50 to 75 percent reduction in seizures.[11]

In a double-blind trial, twenty-four children with epilepsy received vitamin E or a placebo. There was a significant reduction in the number of seizures in ten out of the twelve patients given vitamin E, compared to none of the twelve given a placebo.[12] This study suggests that adjunctive treatment with vitamin E can be of value for people with difficult-to-treat epilepsy. The exact mechanism is unknown, but vitamin E is nontoxic and should perhaps be considered for those whose epilepsy cannot be controlled by conventional treatment. Such therapy might also allow reduction in doses of anticonvulsant medications. In general, begin dosage at 300 IU; increase up to 2,000 IU under nutritional supervision.

Thiamine (Vitamin B₁)

This member of the B vitamin family is essential for healthy nerve cells and proper functioning of the brain and heart. It converts carbohydrates into glucose, the sole energy source for the nervous system. Deficiency may be associated with seizures. Thiamine may be low due to anticonvulsants or eating a diet high in processed foods and sugar. Thiamine is found in whole grains, legumes, poultry, and fish.

Minerals

Although minerals constitute only about 4 or 5 percent of our body weight, every cell of the body depends on minerals for healthy nerve function, as well as for building bones, teeth, tissue, muscle, and blood cells. Minerals belong to two groups: bulk minerals and trace minerals. Bulk minerals, such as calcium and magnesium, are needed in larger amounts than trace minerals, such as manganese and copper. However, trace minerals should be considered just as important because we need to maintain a proper balance of minerals for our bodies to function healthily. On the following pages are a number of minerals that are of particular importance for people with seizures.

Calcium

Calcium is the body's most plentiful mineral. Without a steady supply of calcium, your bones and teeth would not remain hard and your brain wouldn't be able to function properly. Since calcium is especially important in normal nerve transmission, it has been recommended that people with epilepsy supplement their diets with 1,000 to 1,500 mg of calcium daily. Symptoms of calcium deficiency include nervousness, depression, headaches, and insomnia.

Chromium

Chromium is important for maintaining cerebral sugar metabolism. Without chromium, insulin cannot transport glucose from the bloodstream to the cells. No definite guidelines have been established, but trace-mineral experts suggest 200 mcg daily, which is usually obtainable from foods, including legumes, leafy vegetables, whole-grain cereals (except rye and corn), fresh fruit juices, brewer's yeast, and nuts.

Copper

There hasn't been much research on the relationship between copper and seizures. However, one study indicated that a deficiency in copper may cause seizures. Another found that catamenial (associated with menstruation) seizures often involve copper imbalance (either too much or too little). Copper is a strong inducer of free-radical creation, especially when taken in excess.

Magnesium

Magnesium is involved in the body's protein production process. It is necessary for the production of hormones and works in the muscles and the nervous, digestive, reproductive, circulatory, and immune systems. Magnesium deficiency can result in lowered immunity, improper muscle function, and impaired digestion. Without adequate magnesium, your nerves can become ragged and ultrasensitive to pain, and production of new protein is impaired. Magnesium requires adequate amounts of B_6 in order to be absorbed by the tissues. (Testing the blood for magnesium levels is not an accurate way to determine tissue and brain levels of magnesium.)

People with epilepsy have been shown to have significantly lower serum magnesium levels as compared to the general population, with seizure activity correlating with the level of hypomagnesemia. Magnesium has been shown, in uncontrolled trial studies, to be of benefit in the control of seizures. Carl Pfeiffer, M.D., found that a magnesium deficiency induces muscle tremors and convulsive seizures; he reported success in controlling the seizure activity of thirty epileptic patients with 450 mg of magnesium per day.[13]

Dr. Lendon Smith writes:

Magnesium deficiency is especially common among epileptics. Tetany [muscular spasms] and convulsions were first shown to occur in magnesium-deficient rats in 1932. Epileptic convulsions in a physically well-trained man occurred after four hours of continuous exercise in hot conditions. Low serum magnesium was the only biochemical parameter.[14]

Low magnesium greatly enhances sensitivity to the excitotoxic effects of glutamate and aspartate. Magnesium also works with calcium, and our bodies need to have a proper calcium-magnesium ratio. Mildred Seelig, M.D., who has been researching magnesium for more than thirty years, found that alcoholics and diabetics (both groups frequently have seizures) are usually low in magnesium. She believes that we should take in no more than two or three times as much calcium as magnesium.

Recommended daily intake of magnesium is 350 mg, but Gary Null, as well as other nutritionists, believes that 450–650 mg for adults and 500 mg for children may be more appropriate. Good sources of magnesium include green leafy vegetables, nuts, seeds, avocados, and turnips. Whole grains, legumes, organic eggs, raw milk, many fruits, and natural sweeteners such as carob, honey, and blackstrap molasses also contain magnesium.

Manganese

Manganese is a trace mineral that, like magnesium, is active in protein production. It's also essential to the structure of bones, teeth, cartilage, and tendons and necessary for transmitting nerve impulses in your brain. Manganese plays an important role in the metabolism of blood sugar and fats.

The link between epilepsy and manganese was first suggested in 1963 when it was observed in a research study that manganese-deficient rats were more susceptible to seizures than manganese-replete animals and that manganese-deficient animals exhibited an epileptic-like EEG.[15] Low whole blood and hair manganese levels have been found in epileptics, and those with the lowest levels typically having the highest seizure activity.

Yukio Tanaka, M.D., of St. Mary's Hospital in Montreal, Canada, has demonstrated a link between manganese deficiency and convulsions in humans. He also states that pregnant women with a deficiency of manganese may give birth to epileptic children. Pregnant rats consuming a low-manganese diet delivered babies with poorly coordinated movements and a susceptibility to convulsions.

Manganese plays a significant role in cerebral function as it is a critical cofactor for glucose utilization within the neuron, adenylate cyclase activity, and neurotransmitter control. So, optimal central nervous system function requires proper manganese levels. Manganese supplementation may be helpful in controlling seizure activity for some patients.[16] In one study, a boy with seizures that were unresponsive to medications was found to have a blood manganese level that was half the normal value. When supplemented, he had fewer seizures and improvement in gait, speech, and learning.

There is no official recommended daily requirement for manganese, but trace-mineral experts suggest we should include up to 7 mg in our daily diets. Nuts, seeds, and whole grains are excellent sources of manganese that can be found at any grocery or organic-foods store. Green leafy vegetables, broccoli, carrots, potatoes, peas, beans, rhubarb, pineapple, blueberries, raisins, cloves, and ginger, especially if they are grown organically in mineral-rich soil, are also good sources of manganese easily incorporated into our diets.

Selenium

Since selenium and vitamin E function synergistically, both must be taken to correct a deficiency in either. Because studies have shown that people with epilepsy have low levels of selenium, supplementation with selenium and vitamin E results in fewer seizures. Selenium is an excellent antioxidant. (For more information on the importance of vitamin E, see page 117.)

Zinc

Zinc plays an important role in blood sugar balance, protein synthesis, brain function, and the immune system, as well as other aspects of health. Children with epilepsy have been found to have significantly lower levels of serum zinc, especially those with West or Lennox-Gastault syndrome. More important, it appears that people with epilepsy may have an elevated copper-to-zinc ratio. Seizures may be triggered when zinc levels fall, as in the absence of adequate taurine.[17] Although the exact role of zinc, or the copper-to-zinc ratio, is not clearly understood, it appears that anticonvulsants may cause zinc deficiency, either by reducing zinc absorption in the intestines or by causing diarrhea. Therefore, zinc supplementation may be warranted.

The availability of excess zinc, delivered either by dietary supplementation or by injection, has been found to protect against the development of seizures in at least three different animal models of epilepsy.[18]

Amino Acids

Amino acids are the chemical units, or "building blocks," that make up proteins. They combine in various ways to create hundreds of different types of proteins in our bodies. Next to water, protein makes up the greatest portion of our body weight. Amino acids also enable vitamins and minerals to function effectively. In the human body, the liver produces about 80 percent of the amino acids we need, called nonessential amino acids. The remaining 20 percent, essential amino acids, must be obtained from the food we eat. Some amino acids act as neurotransmitters, which can pass through the blood-brain barrier. Then the brain can use them to communicate with nerve cells elsewhere in our bodies.

Carnitine

Carnitine is not an amino acid in the strictest sense; it's actually related to the B vitamins. But because it has a chemical structure similar to that of amino acids, it is usually grouped with them. It helps transport fatty acids into the mitochondria, part of the cell that contains enzymes responsible for the conversion of food into usable energy. Carnitine deficiency is not uncommon in patients with epilepsy. Research has found carnitine levels to be lowest in patients taking valproate, but levels may be low in those taking other anticonvulsants, too. This can be a cause of concern because more than one hundred people have died from valproate-induced hepatic (liver) failure.[19]

About 90 percent of total body carnitine is in muscle tissue, much higher than in the blood, so a normal blood carnitine level reading may be misleading. Symptoms of carnitine deficiency include listlessness, hypoglycemia, heart failure, and muscle weakness. People low in carnitine benefit from supplementation. Many nutritionists believe that acetyl-carnitine has better brain penetration than L-carnitine and also enhances brain levels of acetylcholine.

Dimethylglycine (DMG)

Dimethylglycine (DMG) is formed from betaine in the metabolism of homocysteine to methionine and is a precursor of glycine, a neuroinhibitory amino acid. DMG has also been shown to block induced seizures in rats and mice. Two researchers reported in the *New England Journal of Medicine* a striking decrease in seizure frequency in a patient with long-standing mental retardation when 90 mg of DMG were administered twice daily. Despite treatment with phenobarbital and carbamazepine, the patient had an average of sixteen to eighteen generalized seizures a week, but within one week of starting DMG, seizure frequency dropped to three per week. Two attempts to withdraw the DMG caused dramatic increases in seizure frequency.[20]

It has been suggested that glycine and betaine may act indirectly on glycine metabolism and glycine-mediated neuronal inhibition, may enhance GABA activity, or may simply have a nonspecific effect on biological membranes.

Gamma-Aminobutyric Acid (GABA)

Gamma-aminobutyric acid, as the brain's major inhibitory neurotransmitter, tends to be at lower-than-normal levels in seizure-prone rats and humans with epilepsy. This neurotransmitter has a calming or inhibitory effect on the nervous system. Vitamin B_6 and zinc are necessary for the synthesis of GABA. Little research has been done, but daily supplementation of 500 to 1,000 mg of GABA has been shown to help prevent seizures.

Glutamine

Every cell in the body uses glutamine, particularly the cells in the brain. It's considered a nonessential amino acid, a misleading term because *nonessential* doesn't mean it is unimportant; it means that the body can make it itself.

In the brain, glutamine works to produce excitatory and inhibitory neurotransmitters, primarily glutamate and GABA. Glutamine is also an important source of energy for the nervous system. Cardiovascular function is controlled by the nervous system, and those pathways involved in the neural-heart connection rely on glutamine and GABA. Glutamine is also beneficial for the liver because it cleanses the liver—this assumes an even greater importance when someone is taking anticonvulsants. Glutamine helps prevent hypoglycemia by converting to glucose when blood sugar is low. Some nutritionists recommend supplementation to eliminate sugar and alcohol cravings.

Taurine

Taurine is one of the most abundant amino acids in the body. It is found in the central nervous system and in skeletal muscle and is highly concentrated in the brain and heart. It is an unusual fatty acid (the brain is composed primarily of fatty tissue). Unlike most other amino acids, it prefers to participate in reactions, such as nerve excitability, rather than tissue construction. Taurine is found in mother's milk but not in cow's milk. Animal protein is also a good source of taurine.

Taurine works as an inhibitory neurotransmitter. Like magnesium, taurine affects cell membrane electrical excitability by normalizing potassium flow in and out of heart cells. "Taurine is a stabilizer of membrane excitability and thus could control the onset of epileptic seizures," says Carl Pfeiffer, M.D., former director of the Brain Bio Center at Rocky Hill, New Jersey.

Taurine also has been found to have an effect similar to insulin on blood sugar levels. Taurine helps to stabilize cell membranes and seems to have some antioxidant and detoxifying activity. It helps the movement of potassium, sodium, calcium, and magnesium in and out of cells, which helps generate nerve impulses. Taurine has been used with varying degrees of success in the treatment of a wide variety of conditions, including cardiovascular diseases, high cholesterol, epilepsy and other seizure disorders, macular degeneration, Alzheimer's disease, alcoholism, and cystic fibrosis.[21] Most studies have found that taurine is diminished in the epileptic brain and that it is an anticonvulsant. When genetically susceptible animals are raised on taurine-deficient diets, they develop epilepsy.[22] Transport of taurine can also be impaired in those with epilepsy.

Some studies have shown reduction in seizures when people took 500 mg of taurine three times a day. Other studies have used dosages ranging from 200 mg to 1,500 mg. Some studies have had mixed results, finding that the effects last only temporarily. But Robert Atkins, M.D., in his book *Dr. Atkins' Vita-Nutrient Solution*, writes:

> My patients with epilepsy or similar brain irritability remain free of seizures when they take taurine regularly. Seizures caused by the swelling of brain tissues, such as occurring with brain tumors, are relieved by taurine. . . . Certain excitotoxin chemicals, such as monosodium glutamate and aspartame, lower the body's concentration of taurine, which may be one reason why these food additives are associated with seizure activity.

Dr. Atkins also says some patients have discontinued seizure medication while using taurine.[23]

Acid-Alkaline Balance

When people hear the phrase "balanced diet," they usually think of eating foods from all the basic food groups. But maintaining a proper balance of acid and alkaline (pH) is essential to our health and vitality. The typical American diet is highly acidic; generally, meat, cereals, and junk foods are acidic, whereas fruits and vegetables are alkaline. This helps to explain the popularity of antacid tablets—

they are alkaline and neutralize stomach acid. However, neutralizing stomach acid with pills can result in more digestive problems. According to naturopath Skye Weintraub, even the rate at which you breathe affects the acid-alkaline balance of your body.

The pH ratio in a normal, healthy body is approximately four to one: four parts alkaline to one part acid. Dr. Lendon Smith believes that alkalinity in nerves and muscles is a major factor in epilepsy. He recalls two epileptic patients of his whose blood tests indicated their chemistry was alkaline. Eating more acidic foods (including most fish and meats, most grains, and most nuts), as well as drinking an eight-ounce glass of water containing a teaspoon of vinegar twice a day, helped reduce their seizures.

One naturopath reported that he treated a child who had a seizure each time she ate food that caused her body to become too alkaline. Correcting her pH balance by avoiding certain foods helped reduce her seizures.

Supplements assist the body in digesting and assimilating food, but they are not substitutes for food. And eating unhealthy foods will counteract any potential benefits from vitamin supplements. Most supplements should be taken with meals, and since they are concentrates and devoid of water, a glass of water will help your body digest them. To decide on proper dosages of nutrients, it's always best to consult a nutritionally oriented health practitioner. If your doctor knows little about nutrition, he may consider working with a nutritionist or naturopath.

CHAPTER 8

The Ketogenic Diet

*For the most part, we have our little girl back. Her brain
has been unlocked.*

—TIM COLFER, WHOSE DAUGHTER IS ON THE
KETOGENIC DIET

One of the few alternative treatments that has been accepted by the
medical community, the ketogenic diet alters the body's chemistry
through a very strict diet. Named for the ketones excreted in the
urine during ketosis, this diet contains a ratio of fat calories to protein and carbohydrate calories of three or four to one. It was created
in the 1920s, making it one of the oldest and most effective therapies for preventing or mitigating seizures in children with epilepsy.

Unfortunately, as anticonvulsants became more available in the
1940s and 1950s, the ketogenic diet fell out of favor. But in the past
few years it has experienced a resurgence due to parents' requests for
it. Since studies have demonstrated that a child's ability to extract
ketones from the blood into the brain is four to five times greater
than an adult's, the diet has been used primarily in young children
and teenagers. A few studies on adults are under way. However,

adults have a harder time developing the ketones necessary for the diet to succeed; it is also more difficult for adults to stick to the rigorous diet.

Something Old, Something New

In 1921, Dr. R. M. Wilder, a diabetologist at the Mayo Clinic, came up with a diet that he hoped would prolong the state of ketosis (occurring when the body is forced to burn fat instead of sugar) in diabetics. A stringent, low-calorie diet that is extremely high in fat and low in protein and carbohydrates was further developed at the Mayo Clinic and Johns Hopkins University for children with epilepsy. Studies conducted in the 1930s found that the diet completely controlled seizures in nearly 50 percent of children on the diet and markedly improved seizure control in 75 percent.[1] However, as new antiseizure medications became available in the 1940s and 1950s, the diet fell into disuse.

Researchers at Johns Hopkins University Hospital, including Dr. Samuel Livingstone, Dr. John Freeman, and dietician Millicent Kelly, helped keep the diet alive, refining it for decades. Its biggest boost, though, came from a boy named Charlie.

In 1993, Charlie Abrahams, then just one year old, was diagnosed with Lennox-Gastault syndrome, a rare and often difficult-to-treat form of childhood epilepsy that usually involves several kinds of seizures. He reportedly had up to a hundred seizures a day and medications weren't helping. Charlie's parents, Jim and Nancy, took Charlie to a number of pediatric neurologists, all of whom advised more drugs or brain surgery. His case seemed hopeless.

Jim spent hours researching epilepsy treatments at a medical library. There he read about the ketogenic diet, which had not been mentioned by any of the neurologists who had evaluated Charlie's condition. Although Charlie's neurologist at the time was skeptical, Jim and Nancy insisted that Charlie at least try the diet. Within seventy-two hours of starting the ketogenic diet, Charlie's seizures stopped.

But the Abrahams didn't stop there. In 1994 they started the Charlie Foundation to Cure Pediatric Epilepsy to help other children. In 1997 Jim, a Hollywood director, wrote and directed a television movie, *First Do No Harm*, inspired by their experience with the ketogenic diet. Both efforts have pushed the keto diet into the limelight, inspiring parents to ask their child's neurologist about the diet and helping thousands of children with intractable seizures. They've also raised public consciousness about epilepsy. (For more information on the Charlie Foundation, see Resources.)

Parents whose children are on the keto diet support each other by sharing ideas, questions, innovative recipes (checked by a dietician), and experiences they have. One such group was formed by Elaine Huffman, whose son Michael is on the diet. She founded the Keto Klub, for kids on the diet and their families. She publishes a monthly newsletter for parents and has a keto chat room on the Internet.

What Is the Ketogenic Diet?

The ketogenic diet was originally developed at the Mayo Clinic and Johns Hopkins University Hospital in the 1920s. This high-fat, low-protein and low-carbohydrate diet is devised individually to fit the age, height, and weight of each child. Approximately 90 percent of total calories come from fat, usually in the form of butter, oil, and heavy or whipped cream.

The ketogenic diet is designed to sustain the state of ketosis in the body. Ketosis occurs when the body is forced to burn fat instead of sugar. Ketones, which are left after the fat is burned, build up in the blood and inhibit seizures, although exactly how is unknown.

The diet has been effective with many children who haven't responded to medication. John Freeman, M.D., professor of pediatric neurology at the Johns Hopkins Children's Center at Johns Hopkins University, one of the very few neurologists who has been using this diet, maintains that the keto diet completely controls seizures in more than half of the children who began the diet at Johns Hopkins. Research has backed up his claims. The *Tufts University Health and Nutrition Letter* reported that one-third of children on the ketogenic diet have a significant reduction in seizure incidence, sometimes to the point of becoming seizure free.[2]

The results of the diet's most definitive study to date, which was published in *Pediatrics*, has increased its credibility. The study's research team, led by Dr. Freeman, followed 150 children, ages one to sixteen, for a year on the ketogenic diet. At the start of the study, the children had an average of 410 seizures a month and, on average, had tried six anticonvulsant medications. At the end of the trial year, 55 percent of the original patients remained on the diet. More than half experienced a 50 percent or greater reduction in the number of seizures; 27 percent had a better than 90 percent decrease in seizure frequency.[3]

"Our study shows that despite new and improved anticonvulsant medication on the market," says Dr. Freeman, "the ketogenic diet is still a viable option for children with difficult-to-manage epilepsy." Many neurologists who even a few years ago viewed the ketogenic diet with skepticism are now acknowledging its value.

How Can Fat Stop Seizures?

When glucose reserves are depleted (through fasting, for example), the body can no longer use glucose for energy. This forces the body into a state of ketosis, burning fat faster than it can be completely used, which causes a residue of ketones to build up in the blood and then spill over into the urine. When these ketones build up, they act as a kind of sedative, preventing the sudden disturbances in the electrical functioning of the brain that lead to seizures. Because the aim of the ketogenic diet is to get the body to use fat for energy rather than the usual glucose, carbohydrates and proteins are severely limited. For the diet to successfully control seizures, a child's body must be in a constant state of ketosis.

A whopping 90 percent of calories in this diet comes from fat, including whipped cream, butter, or butter substitutes such as margarine, mayonnaise, and oil. Researchers still don't understand how the diet actually works, but they do know that this diet causes the body to react as though it were fasting. (Management of seizures by fasting and dehydration has been known for centuries. It was even mentioned in the King James Bible, in Matthew 17:14–21 and Mark 9:14–29. But fasting is hardly a permanent solution to seizure control.)

Foods are designated as either K, ketogenic, or AK, antiketogenic. Fats are ketogenic, while carbohydrates (sugars and starches) are antiketogenic. Proteins have a mixed or neutral potential. So whipped cream is good, candy bars are bad, and bacon is so-so. The diet is ordered in terms of a K:AK ratio, which may be five to one, four or five to one, three to one, or two to one. A four-to-one ratio consists of 4 g of fat to 1 g of protein and carbohydrate together. A child will be eating from two to five times as many fat calories as protein and carbohydrate combined.

Because the diet must be tailored to each individual, there isn't a standard set of menus that will apply to all children; the diet is calculated specifically to each child's age, height, weight, and metabolism. Fluid intake is restricted, with children generally allowed one ounce of fluid per pound of body weight. The diet is not nutritionally adequate, so multivitamins and mineral supplements are necessary, particularly calcium and several B vitamins. Everything, including toothpastes, medicine, and vitamins, must be sugar free. Kids on the diet must avoid foods such as pastries, sodas, potato chips, and pretzels. A sample daily meal plan for one child follows:

Breakfast: bacon, a mushroom omelette, and cream

Lunch: celery sticks with peanut butter and cream cheese, lettuce with mayonnaise, sugar-free Jello with cream, and a diet soda

Dinner: part of a chicken breast, broccoli with cheese, lettuce with mayonnaise, whipped cream with one strawberry, and a diet soda

Families often plan meals around the diet. As one mother said in the Keto Klub newsletter, "We have three other children and they all help with the diet." One child said, "I'm a special kid on a special diet!"

Admittedly, because the diet is very rigid and high in fat, it can cause some complications, such as stunted growth, constipation, and high cholesterol. Since studies have shown that a child's early diet programs the genes for later disease, it's possible that this high-fat diet could later lead to the onset of illnesses such as cancer and atherosclerosis, a form of heart disease. Says Dr. Blaylock, "I would suggest that children on the ketogenic diet have a high proportion of extra virgin olive oil as the principal fat, since it reduces atherosclerosis and cancer risk and contains powerful antioxidants."

Getting Started

Children always start the diet in the hospital, where they undergo a two- or three-day fast. Here they are carefully observed for any negative responses to the fasting, such as hypoglycemia, dizziness, dehydration, and seizures. (Most children tolerate this period well, though it seems to be harder on the parents.)

Once the children are excreting a large amount of ketones in their urine, they have achieved ketosis. Then they are gradually introduced to the keto diet and parents are instructed on recipes, measuring food to the gram, and counting calories. The ketogenic diet must never be undertaken without proper medical and nutritional supervision. The risks of an unsupervised diet can include malnutrition, vitamin deficiencies, and chemical imbalances. Dr. Freeman says that several children have died as a result of unsupervised ketogenic diets.

Some children experience a lessening or cessation of seizures immediately upon fasting to reach ketosis. For others, it may take one to three months. Unlike many medications, the diet does not appear to inhibit mental development. Even children who are developmentally delayed or retarded can benefit from the diet; when their seizures cease or are mitigated, they often make developmental progress.

The diet has helped numerous kids whose only options had been multiple medications or brain surgery. One mother said of her four-year-old son, "He is a totally different child. He finally rides a tricycle, and full speech and motor skills have returned." Another child, who averaged fifteen absence seizures a day while taking Tegretol, became medication free and seizure free after a month on the diet.

The ketogenic diet is usually a last resort. It can be used with all forms of epilepsy and can be used with, or in place of, anticonvulsants. Before deciding to use the diet, it might be beneficial to test for food allergies and sensitivities. The average length of time a child is on the diet is two years, and amazingly, after being taken off the diet many children's seizures never return or are limited to just a few. Children on the diet sometimes have seizures—often due to eating prohibited foods. Even eating a cookie or several nuts can eliminate the ketosis and perhaps cause a seizure.

According to Dr. James Wheless, director of the epilepsy-monitoring unit at the University of Texas at Houston, "It is my belief that every pediatric comprehensive epilepsy center should be familiar with the ketogenic diet. Even though physicians perceive the diet as unpalatable and difficult to initiate and maintain . . . the diet is no harder for the physician to initiate than some of our new antiepileptic drugs."

There is another form of the ketogenic diet, called the medium-chain triglycerides (MCT) diet, in which fats are given in the form of an oil. However, according to Dr. Freeman, the MCT diet is not as effective as the keto diet.

Recently, researchers at the University of Southern California have singled out a chemical in the ketogenic diet that has an anticonvulsive effect. The chemical, beta-hydroxybutyrate (BHB), is produced naturally in the body but is produced in larger amounts in people on the ketogenic diet.

Identifying the chemical is the first step toward developing a medication that might replicate its effects. Some parents are uncomfortable about the possibility of replacing the diet with a pill.

Some physicians claim the keto diet works like a drug, and it is true that the diet radically alters a child's biochemistry. But there is a difference between imposing change from outside and imposing change from within. Another question is, if a pill must be bought, will it cost more than food prepared at home? Or would the convenience of not having to weigh food and measure calories be worth the extra cost?

In his book *Seizures and Epilepsy in Childhood* Dr. John Freeman writes:

> Despite anecdotal stories, there is no evidence that food allergies or the elimination diets used to control them play any role in the treatment of epilepsy. . . . Except in rare, specific problems, the addition of other vitamins or mineral supplements to a balanced diet is of NO [emphasis his] documented benefit in the treatment of seizures. . . . There is no evidence that epilepsy is caused by a deficiency of vitamins, minerals, or diet.[4]

Dr. Freeman deserves a lot of credit for keeping this treatment alive, but I think it's wrong to deny the importance of nutrition, especially since the role of food allergies and nutrition with epilepsy is documented. It's odd that a physician whose practice of a diet impugned for so long by most neurologists so ardently rebukes other ways of treating epilepsy. However, he does seem to contradict himself when he writes a few paragraphs later:

> Calcium is a very important mineral for the normal functioning of brain cells, and low levels of calcium can cause

seizures. . . . A deficiency of magnesium, a mineral that interacts with calcium, may cause low blood calcium and, thus, seizures.[5]

It seems the medical establishment has had an easier time accepting the ketogenic diet than other alternative treatments, perhaps because the diet allows doctors to keep a hand in the process. Patients still rely on physicians. The keto diet is now a respectable option, and it has opened the door for other treatments. Now that the ketogenic diet is more accessible, more researched, and gaining in credibility, its success increases the accessibility—and acceptability—of other alternative treatments. Says Elaine Huffman, whose son Michael has benefited greatly from the ketogenic diet, "We all have the right to treatment, no matter how hokey it may seem."

Note: Parents whose children have more than twenty seizures a day and who have not previously been treated with the ketogenic diet may be eligible for a study funded by the National Institutes of Health. Contact Diana Pillas at (410) 955-9100.

CHAPTER 9

The Power of Herbs

We are all healers.
—Susun Weed, author of *Healing Wise*

Herbal medicine is, basically, the use of plants to heal. There is a long tradition of using herbs in the treatment of seizures. But all of the anecdotal history comes from situations where no pharmaceutical drugs have been used. Although most herbs are safe when properly used, scientific research on herbs is still in the elementary stages and potential dangers of herb-drug interactions are not well documented. Because little research has been done on herbs and seizure disorders or on combining synthetic medications with herbs, it is best to read about herbs, discuss taking herbs with your physician, and find an herbalist experienced in working with seizure disorders; ideally, they can work together to supervise your safe journey through herbal treatment. Herbs, which vary in freshness and potency, are available at health-food stores or through mail-order companies. Or you can grow them yourself.

It can be dangerous to give children herbs that are formulated for an adult's size and metabolism. Some companies offer herbal extracts specially for children, but always check with an herbalist before giving children or infants herbs.

Herbal Allies

Herbal remedies have been relied on for centuries. According to the director of the World Health Organization's Traditional Medicine Program, up to 80 percent of the Earth's people still rely on various forms of natural healing. In China, where the use of herbs is an integral part of traditional medicine, more than five hundred different plants are "official drugs." In Germany, one-third of graduating physicians have taken courses in herbal medicine.

Compared to their pharmaceutical counterparts, herbs exhibit a slower and deeper action. Herbs have more than one chemical in them, so when you take an herb, you may be getting a number of active components. Additionally, herbs serve not only as medicine but also as nutritious foods, with many herbs being rich in vitamins and minerals. That's one way herbs help heal our bodies, while drugs don't. Drugs control the symptoms; that is their benefit and their limitation.

Nobody is sure just how herbs work. Kathi Keville, an herbal educator from Nevada City, California, says:

All of us have theories. Nobody knows for sure. What is clear is that plants produce complex compounds of chemicals, and one theory contends that when you use a botanical remedy instead of a drug containing only a synthesized version of the plant's active ingredient, you're actually using a highly complex package of drugs. This bundle of plant chemicals then works together to produce a medicine that is more than the sum of its active ingredients.[1]

Green Pharmacy

There are two kinds of herbs. First, there are tonic herbs, which have a strengthening and normalizing effect on some or all of the body systems. Most of them are *adaptagenic*, meaning they are able to bring the system back into harmony, whether the needed influence is to increase or decrease a function. For instance, in cardiovascular therapy, tonic herbs can increase or decrease blood pressure as needed. In the case of nervous system tonic herbs, they can have an excitatory or inhibitory effect, as needed.

Second, there are herbs that are used for one and only one purpose and have a one-directional influence. Most herbalists suggest that anyone using prescription drugs to treat an epileptic condition should start with the tonic herbs. Nancy Nina, R.N., suggests that individuals choose tonic herbs that have all of the properties of the herb present, both active and inactive, and avoid using guaranteed potency and standardized extract herbs. These latter formulas have been altered so that some of the naturally occurring elements in the plant are in greater proportion to others.

How to Begin Taking Herbs

When introducing herbs, it's prudent to move slowly and gradually. It's best to take the herbs traditionally used in the treatment of convulsive disorders as teas rather than in tinctures or capsules, at least at first, because teas are absorbed more slowly than tinctures or capsules. Then, when you want to take more, use a capsule or tincture. It is always advisable to check with your health-care practitioner before taking herbs, particularly if you are also taking prescription drugs.

People with seizure disorders who are taking anticonvulsant medications should avoid the use of alcohol. Since most tinctures are in an alcoholic base, tinctures should probably be avoided when you first start taking herbs. If you do use a tincture, look for one made with glycerine—children should take herbs made with glycerine. If you can't find glycerine tinctures, the alcohol can be removed by putting the desired amount of the tincture in a cup and pouring a small amount of boiling water over the tinctured herb. This evaporates the alcohol, leaving the desired properties of the herb intact.

Nancy Nina believes that another reason to avoid the use of tinctures when introducing herbs into the body is that the concentrations of the herb are greater in the tinctures and they get into the system faster. You may want to slowly introduce one or more of these plant allies into your body. Nina suggests that herbs be introduced one at a time, slowly and cautiously, keeping track of your response to its presence in your body.

Be sure to keep a record of when you started taking a particular herb, how much you took, and how you responded to it. When you are comfortable with one herb, confident that your body can tolerate it and that it is all right to take with your prescription drug, make note of that and try a different antiseizure herb. Follow the same introductory process, documenting dosages and responses. Many people prefer to use any one herb continuously for a month or two and then to stop taking it, so they can assess how it has affected their body and whether or not it is still of benefit to continue its use. There is no need to slowly taper off the herbs when stopping one and starting another. In this way, you can gain familiarity and confidence with a whole family of herbal allies.

Never abruptly stop taking medication. According to Dr. Andrew Weil, "Even if a person who never had any problems with seizures were to start taking these drugs and then suddenly stop them, they would have seizures." His recommendation is to slowly introduce the herb of choice—he suggests valerian—while continuing to take medication. Only after fully establishing a strong presence of the herb in your system would he suggest a very gradual diminishing of the dose of the antiseizure medication, and then only under the supervision of a qualified medical practitioner. In using herbs, says Dr. Weil, "the goal is not to eliminate the drugs totally (although I have seen occasional patients succeed at that) but to reduce them to a level you can live with, so that you can enjoy normal alertness and still not have seizures."

In addition, since the goal in treating seizure disorders is to reduce the excitability of the brain, Dr. Weil recommends eliminating all stimulants, including tobacco, coffee, tea, cola, and chocolate.

Bridging Herbal and Allopathic Medicine

Below are a number of herbs that reportedly help people with epilepsy. Because pharmaceuticals can sometimes have harmful interactions with herbs, I've also listed the known effects of the interactions of anticonvulsive medications and herbs used for epilepsy.

Valerian   During the late 1500s, valerian's popularity grew after an Italian physician claimed he cured himself of epilepsy by using it. In the United States, colonists discovered several Native American tribes using the pulverized roots of valerian to treat wounds. Their use of the herb brought it to the attention of physician Samuel Thomson, who called valerian "the best nervine [tranquilizer] known." Valerian entered the U.S. pharmacopoeia as a tranquilizer in 1820 and remained there until 1942. It was listed in the *National Formulary*, a pharmaceutical guide, until 1950. Research has shown the ability of valerian to bind GABA-receptors. Sedation in the central nervous system is primarily mediated through these receptors. According to Michael Castleman, author of *The Healing Herbs*, a number of animal studies suggest valerian has anticonvulsant effects. Dr. Weil suggests using nonalcoholic tincture of valerian as a natural, mild depressant. Take one dropperful in a little water three or four times a day. Store valerian away from light.

Herbalist Daniel Mowrey, author of *Herbal Tonic Therapies*, says that although valerian is generally used for its sedative and tranquilizing effect on the central nervous system, it has a stimulating effect in some individuals. It does not react with alcohol and does not leave one with a groggy, drugged hangover.

Side effects: Research has indicated minimal side effects using valerian. A small percentage of persons using the extract may experience mild, transient stomach upset. Some herbalists caution that long-term uninterrupted use may lead to depression.

Contraindications: Persons currently taking sedative drugs or antidepressants should take valerian only under the supervision of a health-care professional. European pharmacopeias list no contraindication to use valerian root during pregnancy and childbirth.[2]

Drug interactions: No harmful effects are known.

Skullcap   This herb reportedly relaxes the central nervous system. Skullcap is one of the herbs many herbalists recommend for the treatment of convulsive disorders. It is available as a dried herb and in an alcohol solution.

Side effects: Skullcap may have an effect on hormones.

Contraindications: No known medical conditions preclude its use.

Drug interactions: No interactions have been reported. No harmful effects are known if you are pregnant or breast-feeding.

Black Cohosh   This member of the buttercup family is beneficial because it aids in controlling the central nervous system and has a calming effect. Studies on mutagenicity and carcinogenicity have proved negative. A study on long-term administration (six months)

An Herbal Success Story

Rosemary Gladstar, an herbalist and author of several books on herbalism, developed an herbal program for Jennifer, her stepdaughter. Jennifer began having seizures when she was an infant and had seizures all through her childhood. To control her seizures, her doctors first tried phenobarbital, but phenobarbital stunted her growth. Then she tried Dilantin, which made her sleepy. She switched to Tegretol, but she felt tired all the time, an apparent side effect of the medication. With Gladstar's help and Jennifer's physician monitoring her progress, she began herbal therapy. This included ginkgo, gotu kola tinctures, and vitamin B supplements.

"It gave me a lot more energy," Jennifer said. She stayed on the program, which included dietary and lifestyle changes, before slowly discontinuing it. As a result, her physician was able to lower her dosage of Tegretol by nearly half.[5]

to rats failed to show chronic toxicity at about ninety times the human dose equivalent. These findings concur with more than sixty years of safe clinical experience, especially in Germany. [3]

Side effects: No health hazards or side effects are known in conjunction with the proper administration of designated therapeutic dosages. An intake of very high dosage (5 g) or an extract (12 g) can cause vomiting, headache, dizziness, and lowered blood pressure. Adverse side effects at a normal dosage include gastric discomfort.[4]

Contraindications: Because of its hormonelike effect (it's often used to treat menopausal disorders), check with your doctor before taking during pregnancy or while breast-feeding. There are no known medical conditions that preclude the use of this herb.

Drug interactions: None have been reported.

Gotu Kola   Originally an Asian medication, gotu kola is used in the Far East for a number of problems, including asthma, insomnia, depression, epilepsy, and heart problems.

Side effects: High doses have been known to cause nausea. Sedation and skin rashes are also possible.

Contraindications: Not recommended during pregnancy or breast-feeding. No other medical conditions preclude its use.

Drug interactions: No drug interactions have been reported.

Ginkgo Biloba   The active compounds in ginkgo extract improve circulation and protect nerve cells from harm when deprived of oxygen. These ingredients also appear to have an antioxidant effect, sparing brain tissue from damage caused by free radicals. Because the active ingredients are limited to minute quantities in natural ginkgo leaves, only concentrated ginkgo extract is really effective. Ginkgo extract is produced in liquid and solid forms, often as 40 mg tablets. Tea made from ginkgo leaves, as in traditional Chinese medicine, is considered too weak to be effective.

Discussing tonic herbs for the nervous system, herbalist Daniel Mowrey suggests that ginkgo biloba and Siberian ginseng may be of benefit because they act to increase cerebral blood circulation and thus improve the oxygenation of the brain. These tonic herbs can be introduced at any time, without concern for their interaction with the anticonvulsant properties of the pharmaceuticals, inasmuch as their properties are not synergistic. It should be mentioned that the ginkgo does have anticlotting properties, so it is important to be cautious in its use if there are any bleeding problems or if you are taking any other anticlotting drugs or herbs, such as aspirin, coumadin, heparin, dong quai, gotu kola, turmeric, or large doses of garlic.

Side effects: Use can occasionally lead to spasms, cramps, and mild digestive problems. On rare occasions, allergic skin reactions may occur.

Contraindications: Anyone with bleeding problems should avoid using this herb.

Drug interactions: None have been recorded.

Vervain   Sometimes listed as blue vervain, this herb has been shown to be especially helpful for absence seizures, particularly if triggered by menstrual changes.[6]

Side effects: Studies demonstrating the effects on the immune system have not been conclusive. Animal studies have shown an increase in urinary output and effects on salivation and lactation.

Contraindications: This herb should not be taken during pregnancy or when breast-feeding.

Drug interactions: No known drug interactions.

Marijuana   Until the middle part of this century, *Cannabis sativa* enjoyed a long and respectable history as a medicinal agent. As early as 2737 B.C., the plant was included in the pharmacopoeia of the Chinese emperor Shen Nung. But in the 1960s and 1970s it lost its respectability when it became a popular recreational drug. Despite that, in a November 15, 1994, petition to Health and Human Services Secretary Donna Shalala, the Federation of American Scientists (FAS) called on the federal government to research marijuana's medicinal use. The FAS pointed out that whole cannabis is already in clinical use by patients suffering a variety of illnesses, including epilepsy.

Under California's Proposition 215, passed several years ago, it is legal for any "seriously ill" California adult to obtain marijuana on the recommendation of a physician. Valerie Corral has had seizures since being injured in an auto accident twenty-four years ago. Her doctors put her on a regimen of drugs that only partly controlled her grand mal seizures. After her husband read an article about a study claiming marijuana smoke controlled seizures in laboratory animals, she tried it and says her seizures stopped. She grows marijuana in her home garden, and she says marijuana is the only drug she uses, taking "a puff or two" whenever she senses the aura that many epileptics experience in the moments before a seizure; she claims that, without fail, it always averts a seizure. The mayor of Santa Cruz, California, recently honored Corral by proclamation in appreciation of her work growing marijuana and giving it free to indigent patients through her nonprofit Wo/Men's Alliance for Medical Marijuana (WAMM).[7]

Side effects: Although marijuana has not been proved to be physically addictive, psychological dependence may develop. Other possible side effects include confusion, panic reaction, fear, and a sense of helplessness. Clinical evidence suggests that long-term use may produce subtle cognitive impairments in memory, attention span, and the ability to organize complex information.

Contraindications: This herb should not be used during pregnancy or when breast-feeding.

Drug interactions: No reported drug interactions, but further research is needed.

Other Helpful Herbs   Other tonic herbs traditionally used in convulsive disorders include passion flower, lobelia (in large doses it may induce vomiting), and mistletoe (to be used in small doses, cautiously). Herbalist Susun Weed says oats and oatstraw help nourish and strengthen the nerves and regulate the nervous system. Even organic oats and oatmeal can be beneficial. She also recommends violet for epileptic memory loss.

Kava kava may also be useful, but apparently it is not sufficiently active to control seizure conditions on its own.[8] Saiko-keishi-to, a Chinese herbal medicine made from a combination of nine botanicals, was reported to have dramatic therapeutic effects on difficult cases of epilepsy that had been unsuccessfully treated with conventional allopathic anticonvulsants.[9]

This is a very brief overview of some useful, and perhaps controversial, herbs for treating epilepsy. Herbs should be used as part of an overall program that includes proper nutrition, adequate sleep, and exercise. If you're interested in learning more, many excellent books on medicinal herbs are available at bookstores and the public library. Whether your aim is to discontinue or lower medication or to simply improve your overall health, always consult an experienced herbalist or nutritionist before you begin herbal therapy—it's unwise to take medicinal herbs without supervision. A reputable health-care professional will never lower dosage or discontinue an anticonvulsant medication until you have been taking the herbs for a sustained period of time.

PART III

Listening to Your Body

Controlling Your Brain Waves

Breath controls brain waves.
—ROBERT FRIED, PH.D.

Stress is a leading cause of seizures. The stress response is the body's primitive fight-or-flight response to danger, whether real or imagined. In preparing to either fight or flee the proverbial saber-toothed tiger, the stress response in humans tenses the muscles and constricts the blood vessels. It also triggers the release of adrenalin and cortisol. These two hormones can have deleterious effects on the body if they are repeatedly activated and can aggravate seizures.

However, most of the stress we encounter today is mental anguish and fear, leaving our bodies in a state of physical tension that leads to decreased energy, fatigue, and lowered immunity. As a preventive measure and as a treatment, relaxation can be an important therapy, as it combats stress and anxiety and strengthens the body's resistance to illness. To relax effectively, our minds should be in the present, not worrying about the past or future, and we need to breathe deeply and slowly. Often when we think we are relaxing, our muscles remain tense and we have not "turned off" mentally.

Of course, everyone's life has stressful features, but we need to distinguish between the healthy stress of job challenges or school demands when we are stimulated and unhealthy stress, in which we feel overwhelmed and powerless. By learning to relax our bodies and identify our stressors (even boredom is a kind of stress), we can avoid those particular stressors or learn how to deal with them. Helping us to distinguish the differences and to deal with both kinds effectively are a number of body therapies, such as biofeedback, progressive relaxation, yoga, meditation, exercise, and simple relaxation "stress busters." These help rid our bodies of tension before it builds up, mostly by teaching us to breathe deeply.

Breathing deeply from the diaphragm comes naturally to healthy babies. Unfortunately, many of us lose this natural capacity when we get older and acquire poor breathing habits. Our mind, body, and spirit work in tandem. One of the body's automatic reactions to stress is rapid, shallow breathing. Breathing slowly and deeply is one of the ways to turn off the stress reaction and turn on the relaxation response. This accomplishes two things: (1) your whole body relaxes, and (2) the flow of oxygen to your brain increases.

Biofeedback

In the first chapter, I mentioned my invaluable experience with biofeedback: once realizing I was a shallow breather, I then consciously learned to breathe deeply. You may find nothing natural about hooking yourself up to a biofeedback machine, and I suppose that's true. But it is a useful tool. Dr. John Basmajian, a founding father of biofeedback, defined it as "the technique of using equipment (usually electronic) to reveal to human beings some of their internal physiologic events, normal and abnormal, in the form of visual and auditory signals in order to teach them to manipulate these otherwise involuntary or unfelt events by manipulating the displayed signals."[1]

Electroencephalogram (EEG) biofeedback measures brain wave activity. This information is then fed into a computer, which translates the patterns on the screen; many have devices that emit audible tones when the person gets into a relaxed state. The machine measures how relaxed your body is by "feeding back" physiological information that the body is giving out via the electrodes pasted to your scalp—information that would be extremely difficult to measure otherwise. Sessions generally last from forty-five minutes to an hour. An entire treatment program can last from ten to fifty sessions or more, depending on the individual's condition.

There are four kinds of brain waves:

- Beta: alert, concentrating, perhaps anxious.
- Alpha: awake and relaxed. Few seizures occur in this state. Not surprisingly, many people with epilepsy have little alpha activity in their EEGs.
- Theta: drowsy, as before you fall asleep. Alpha and theta rhythms offer larger fluctuations of energy than beta. Many people with epilepsy have a lot of theta waves and this state is thought to induce seizures.
- Delta: produced when you sleep.

The alpha brain wave state is the most desirable. As Donna Andrews of the Andrews/Reiter clinic in Santa Rosa, California, says, "Alpha waves are the antithesis of a seizure."

Researchers have trained many people with epilepsy, especially those whose seizures are triggered by stress, to increase brain wave states, usually alpha, to improve control over seizures. Once people have learned to bring on the desired brain waves, they know how it feels and can do it on their own.

Neurofeedback

Neurofeedback is a form of biofeedback that displays a person's brain waves on a computer screen and helps that person to control them. So far, there are no large-scale scientifically controlled studies. Joel Lubar, Ph.D., a psychologist who in 1979 established the Southeastern Biofeedback and Neurobehavioral Institute in Knoxville, Tennessee, has treated about fifty patients with epilepsy, half of whom were able to reduce their seizure rate by about 50 percent or more. "Neurofeedback works best for seizures that have a motor component," says Dr. Lubar, "including tonic-clonic, myoclonic, atonic-akinetic, and partial complex. It is less effective for absence seizures."[2]

Hyperventilation

Biofeedback has been used successfully for a number of conditions, from migraine headaches to addiction. EEG biofeedback has been experimented with for several decades. Barry Sterman, Ph.D., from the School of Medicine at UCLA, has done many experiments using EEG biofeedback. He developed a sensimotor (SMR) system that helps people learn to control the excitability that triggers seizures along the brain's motor pathways. Findings published in the *New Age Journal* show a 60 percent seizure-reduction rate in 70 percent of his patients who were resistant to anticonvulsant medications.[3]

The work of Dr. Sterman and a number of other researchers stemmed from the belief that the reduction of seizures was due to changing electrical activity in the brain. Others, like Dr. Robert Fried, held that seizures were metabolical by enlarging blood vessels, blowing off carbon dioxide, and hyperventilating.

As far back as 1928, says Dr. Fried, William Lennox, M.D., observed that disordered breathing was a common feature among those who had epilepsy. In 1946, he and Dr. E. Gibbs stated:

Considering all those links between CO_2 and epilepsy, namely: (1) the influence of carbon dioxide on the EEG, (2) the abnormal values of carbon dioxide in arterial and jugular blood of patients with petit mal and grand mal, and (3) the abnormal variation of CO_2 preceding grand mal seizures in such a way as to indicate a causal relationship, we may conclude that CO_2 plays a significant role in the etiology of epileptic convulsions.[4]

But even though other researchers have also concluded that seizures arise from a complex metabolic state, "neuro-electrical theories of brain neurons run amok," as Dr. Fried puts it, have prevailed. His research, he says, has been "based on the theory that epilepsy is a disorder of blood flow and brain-cell metabolism, rather than simply a disturbance of brain electrical activity. That is why my emphasis is on breathing. It was intended to restore brain blood flow by increasing brain blood-vessel diameter constricted by the effects of hyperventilation."[5]

When we hyperventilate, we breathe fast, blowing off carbon dioxide, which carries out wastes and toxins, but which the blood platelets need in a certain amount. By breathing too fast we deprive the blood of the carbon dioxide it needs. And carbon dioxide influences nerve-cell function and cerebral electrical activity, which is also why hyperventilating can reduce blood flow to the heart and brain. Dr. Fried believes he is on the right track because most studies of seizures no longer look at EEGs but various brain "scans" of blood flow.

Participants in his studies have experienced significant reduction in seizure activity. In one study, ten people with idiopathic epilepsy and varying kinds of seizures reported an average of fifty-six seizures per month at the beginning of the study. At the end of the first month of biofeedback training, using breathing methods adapted from various yoga techniques, their seizure frequency

dropped to an average of seven seizures per month, then to four
seizures per month. Participants stayed in the program for at least
seven months.[6]

"We did not observe a single instance," Dr. Fried says, "in
which persons presenting with idiopathic epilepsy did not show
moderate to severe chronic hyperventilation. The control group contained a number of people who had moderate to severe hyperventilation, but did not have seizures."[7] (The fact that some who
hyperventilated did not have seizures indicates that their brains
could handle the blood-vessel constriction.) He adds that in one
study he conducted, many of the participants ultimately discovered
their "food triggers"—the foods that affected their seizure frequency—which helped to raise their seizure threshold.

In a study conducted at the Andrews/Reiter Epilepsy Research
Program, 83 percent of patients with complex partial epilepsy
achieved complete control of their seizures by the end of treatment.
The younger the patients were when they started having seizures,
the more sessions they needed, as did those people who experienced
more frequent seizures. But even the people who had the lowest rate
of control at the beginning of the study achieved 67 percent seizure
control.[8]

Biofeedback practitioners recommend that it be used in conjunction with other relaxation techniques, such as deep breathing,
progressive relaxation, and visualization. Dr. Andrews uses biofeedback as one part of overall behavioral conditioning, which includes
nutrition and lifestyle issues. "A seizure is a learned response," she
says. "What we teach our patients is to sense the brain changing
itself. Biofeedback is only a small portion. People realize how to connect how they think with what they feel." She said she has helped
children, the youngest only eight months old. "And I did it by teaching the parents how to hold the baby. The parent-child symbiosis is
so intense a parent can change a child's brain waves."

Progressive Relaxation

Most of us don't realize how tensely we hold ourselves. Progressive relaxation is based on the theory that tensing a muscle and then releasing that tension helps a person become aware of unnecessary muscle tension and contributes to reduction of anxiety throughout the body—and ultimately promotes deep breathing. In three American studies of the effectiveness of progressive relaxation in reducing seizures, it was reported that 88 percent of the participants experienced some seizure reduction with a median reduction rate of 49 percent.[9] A study conducted at Northwestern University found that people with uncontrolled seizures could reduce the frequency of their seizures by nearly 50 percent by practicing progressive relaxation exercises daily.[10]

Progressive muscular relaxation is a three-step technique. (See page 160.) First, you tense a muscle and notice how it feels, then you release the tension and pay attention to that feeling. Then you concentrate on the difference between the two sensations. This can be done sitting or lying down, and it takes only about fifteen minutes. For best results, practice this technique in a quiet, relaxing atmosphere. You could also use creative visualization during this time, imagining you are in a beautiful, peaceful setting. Imagine that your brain and your entire body are functioning in harmony and you are totally healthy.

The Benefits of Exercise

Our bodies were designed to be active, to move. Unfortunately, many children with epilepsy are discouraged from vigorous exercise and play, and they become sedentary. Often we were told by family and physicians to avoid physical activities because they could be strenu-

A Guided Exercise

Lie comfortably on your back or sit in a comfortable chair in a quiet room. As you tense each muscle, inhale, and as you gradually release it, exhale.

1. Clench your toes tightly as you breathe in. Hold your breath and the tension for as long as possible. Then relax and exhale.
2. Flex your right foot. Hold. Relax. Flex your left foot. Hold, then relax and exhale.
3. Tense the calf muscles in your right leg. Hold. Relax and exhale. Tense the calf muscles in your left leg. Hold. Relax.
4. Tense your kneecaps. Hold. Relax. Take a few deep breaths.
5. Raise your right leg about six inches off the floor and tighten your thigh. Hold. Relax and breathe out. Raise your left leg about six inches off the floor. Hold. Relax.
6. Tighten your buttocks. Hold. Relax.
7. Take a deep breath and pull your abdomen in to harden it. Relax. Take a few deep breaths.
8. Make a tight fist with your right hand. Hold. Relax. Make a tight fist with your left hand. Hold. Relax.
9. Bend the elbow of your right arm and point it to the ceiling, tensing both upper and lower arm. Hold. Relax. Repeat with your left arm. Hold. Relax. Take a few deep breaths.
10. Raise your shoulders up to your ears. Hold. Let them drop. Relax.
11. Raise your eyebrows. Hold. Relax.
12. Squeeze your eyes shut. Hold. Relax. Take a few deep breaths.
13. Smile, pulling back the corners of your mouth. Hold. Relax.
14. Drop your jaw and stick out your tongue. Hold. Relax.

ous and trigger seizures. Ironically, seizures while exercising are rare, and overall, exercise helps reduce seizures. Studies of individual patients indicate that sensible physical exercise does not generally precipitate seizures.[11]

Whereas adults view exercise as an ancillary aspect of life—making time for it when we can—children love to be active. Indeed, play and exercise help keep their bodies toned, but activity is also important for the neuromuscular development of their bodies, coordination, and certainly, self-esteem. If children can't play the sports that they love, particularly with other children, they feel limited, which may extend to other aspects of their well-being, making them afraid to push themselves in other endeavors, too. Fear, especially among parents, often leads to overprotection of children with epilepsy, who then feel isolated and restricted. Studies show that exercise improves self-esteem and social integration regardless of seizure control.

The major concern regarding epilepsy and sports participation is that a head injury in a child who has epilepsy could trigger seizures or worsen the amount or duration of seizures. Thus, it is important to understand the relationship between head trauma and epilepsy. One study found the majority of seizures in children occur within twenty-four hours after the trauma. Seizures caused by head injuries are most likely to occur within two years of an accident.

In the past, school administrators have sometimes discouraged children with epilepsy from participating in school sports or gym class. However, federal law now requires that recipients of federal funds, including schools, do not discriminate on the basis of medical disability in their programs.

Balancing Act

In a study of twenty-six children with epilepsy, twenty of the children (77 percent) had fewer epileptic discharges during ten minutes of vigorous cycling.[12] Still, the mechanisms responsible for EEG improvement during exercise are unclear. While hyperventilation is used during EEG recording to increase epileptiform activity, paradoxically, compensatory hyperventilation during exercise improves the EEG. Hyperventilation during exercise, a response to an increasing oxygen demand, prevents hypercapnia, or excessive carbon dioxide in the blood. Hyperventilation during sedentary EEG recording causes respiratory alkalosis with resultant cerebral asoconstriction and hypoxia. Beta endorphin release during exercise may also improve the EEG.[13] Lastly, the increased attention and awareness required during exercise may confer antiepileptic effects. Some researchers have speculated that this increased mental concentration may reduce seizure frequency, but how increased awareness might protect against seizures is not known.

Overall fitness and a feeling of well-being have been shown to help reduce seizure frequency in children and adults. Regular exercise can also alleviate bouts of depression. In a study conducted in the University of Alabama at Birmingham's department of psychology, exercise had a proven positive effect on 133 people with epilepsy. Those who did aerobic exercise at least three times a week for twenty minutes or more reported less stress and fewer emotional problems in general.

However, most antiepileptic medications have side effects that may cause fatigue and lethargy. Others have side effects such as blurred or double vision, concentration difficulty, and impaired coordination that can also hinder performance. For example, phenobarbital and topiramate (Topamax) are thought to impair concentration, while carbamazepine (Tegretol) and phenytoin (Dilantin) may cause impaired coordination.[14]

It's not quite clear what effect brain surgery has on physical exercise. A general rule of thumb for patients being considered for or recovering from surgery is to initiate an exercise program gradually and avoid contact sports, such as football or ice hockey. Preventing head trauma is essential.

Children and Sports

Children who have reliable auras and those who have nocturnal seizures, say most experts, may participate in most activities with supervision. However, contact sports, aviation sports, and unsupervised water sports must be avoided. Those who have more frequent or uncontrolled seizures should be more cautious when choosing sports; they require supervision and safety precautions on the playing field. Sports such as gymnastics, horseback riding, mountain climbing, and the like are generally frowned on for those with epilepsy. However, in the case of horseback riding, many children

Why Exercise?

Regular exercise has these proven benefits:
- improves concentration and alertness
- increases heart efficiency
- improves circulation to the brain
- promotes sounder sleep
- improves digestion and controls appetite
- increases body confidence, overall physical fitness, and stamina
- helps reduce stress, anxiety, boredom, frustration, and depression (people with epilepsy are especially prone to depression)
- helps reduce seizures
- increases exposure to sunlight, which contains vitamin D

who love horses benefit greatly from the relationship between horse and human, as well as a sense of control as a rider. Helmets must always be worn, and children must be supervised.

Most physicians would prefer that a child with epilepsy play tennis rather than soccer. On the other hand, they recognize the psychological damage that can result when youngsters set their heart on playing a particular sport and are told they can't play it because they have epilepsy. In such situations, the psychological benefits of playing may be greater than the physical risks. Common sense should always prevail, and the decision to pursue a particular activity should be based on discussions among athlete, physician, and coach, if there is one.

Let people know what they should do in the event that a seizure occurs. If your child has epilepsy, it is important to tell school administrators, gym instructors, and camp counselors, along with what to do in case your child has a seizure. Otherwise, they'll be taken totally by surprise, which may prevent them from providing the best care.

Athletes of all ages can be inspired by Amber Webster of Chester, Vermont, who despite having epilepsy is active on her high school's cross-country track team and the wrestling team. And by eighteen-year-old Raizel Weinberg of Eugene, Oregon, who says, "I don't let seizures tell me what to do. By being positive and not letting seizures stop me from doing things, I have finally made myself get out and have fun—out in the community, with friends, or just by myself. I enjoy playing my violin and I love the outdoors, camping, going on long bike rides, and hiking." And by cyclist Marion Clignet, a 1996 Olympic silver medalist. "If you let epilepsy get in the way," she says, "it will. But it can't get in your way unless you let it. Epilepsy is no excuse for not getting out there and pursuing your dreams."[15]

If a Seizure Occurs

If someone has a seizure, the most important task is to protect that person from self-injury. This includes helping the person lie down, clearing the area of dangerous objects, loosening all clothing, and rolling the person over on his or her side. Seizures usually stop after a few minutes; if not, call an ambulance.

How soon after a seizure can a child return to play? There is no specific waiting period. Again, common sense should prevail. If the seizure was the first one, a thorough neurological assessment is necessary to determine the cause. If not, the child can return to an activity whenever he or she feels ready. Exercise rarely induces a seizure and, in fact, may help to reduce the frequency of seizures and help to alleviate parents' fears.

If as an adult you're not sure which type of exercise you'd like to do, a good place to start is with a class at a local community college or an adult education program. Not only will you get a sense of how to do the exercise, but exercising with other people will provide support and discipline.

Here are some tips to keep in mind before beginning an exercise program:

1. Identify what you believe are advantages and disadvantages of exercise for you.
2. Discuss your intentions with your physician and a coach, if there is one.
3. List any obstacles you foresee getting in the way of your exercise intentions; for example, worries about a seizure, clumsiness, improper equipment.
4. Choose the kind of exercise you think you'd enjoy. If exercise isn't enjoyable, you won't stick to it.

5. Plan exercise into your schedule and make it a priority. As one doctor has said, "If you're too busy to exercise, then your life is way too busy."

6. Remember: your intent is relaxation, muscle tone, and a feeling of overall well-being.

7. It's important to maintain adequate hydration, avoid overexertion, and ensure adequate sleep and nutrition. Keep water bottles and snacks, such as nuts, granola, or energy bars, available. (Read the labels—many energy bars and drinks contain a lot of refined sugar or high-fructose corn syrup.)

Stress Busters

Vigorous exercise isn't the only kind of movement that benefits the body and mind. Below are a few gentle mind-body workouts that have enormous potential to increase energy and tranquility.

Hatha Yoga

Developed by Indian monks thousands of years ago, yoga consists of a series of postures, called *asanas*. Many of the breathing exercises focus on the intake of *prana*, or life energy. These can be practiced as a series of physical exercises that create peace of mind and relax the body.

Yoga can reduce stress, and the stretching exercises help you understand the difference between feeling tense and feeling relaxed. Relaxation, deep breathing, and postures that massage inner organs can also help with digestive disorders. Certain asanas, such as the shoulder stand and the pose of tranquility, are especially beneficial to the nervous system. Although taking yoga classes with a practitioner is beneficial, videotapes are also available.

Meditation

Traditionally, just about every culture has had a form of meditation. Meditating induces restfulness and peace. Heart rate and blood pressure drop, while blood flow to the brain increases and brain waves switch to alpha rhythm, an indication of relaxation. This deep relaxation dampens the stress response.

Meditation has proved to be beneficial for people with seizures. In one study, researchers found that those who practiced a form of yoga meditation experienced about a third fewer seizures after three months, compared to a control group that showed no improvement.[16] In another study, adults whose seizures were not controlled by medication practiced meditation for twenty minutes a day for one year. Participants showed a significant reduction in seizure frequency and duration. This reduction greatly increased after five to six months of continuous practice.[17]

When you meditate, sit cross-legged in a quiet spot and focus on your breathing. Many people have a mantra, or a word they repeat over and over. If you prefer, you can count your breaths. It's not necessary to take a class in meditation, but reading about the different postures and ways to focus your mind is helpful.

Tai Chi

This ancient practice features extended and natural postures, slow and even motions, and curved, flowing lines of movement. Tai chi motions are described, for example, as follows: "While making a stride, it is as quietly as a cat walks." The movements are gentle and slow, but well-balanced and steady; the breathing deep and even, while the mind is tranquil yet alert. I've recently started taking tai chi classes, and though I feel very clumsy, I'm drawn to its grace, tranquility, and gentleness while feeling aerated afterward.

To learn all of the movements, you'll need to attend classes with a tai chi instructor, available at adult education classes. Children may perform gentle exercises, such as yoga or tai chi. (Full contact karate is not recommended.)

Stretching and Yawning

Quick and easy, stretches and yawns are superb ways to relieve physical and mental stress. Unfortunately, we tend to associate yawns with boredom, so we usually stifle our yawns. But try a yawn deluxe: Open your mouth, lift your arms overhead, and stretch the shoulders and back, enabling the chest to widen and the lungs to open up, making room for incoming oxygen. This process sends fuel to fatigued muscles, especially the brain.

"Yawns flush out and cleanse your lungs, as do sighs," says Rafael Pelayo, M.D., a neurologist at the Sleep Disorders Clinic and Research Center at Stanford University. He has studied yawns and sighs and believes both reflexes to be "interchangeable."[18]

Lilias Folan, a yoga instructor and author of *Yoga and Your Life*, believes that sighs are "the body's way of flushing out the stress caused by pent up feelings of frustration. Which is why yoga instructors exhort students to breathe out distracting thoughts and emotions—and then breathe in good, cleansing oxygen."[19]

Merging Musicology with Neurology

One of the world's oldest medical documents, the Eber Papyrus (dated 1500 B.C.), prescribed incantations that Egyptian physicians chanted to heal the sick. Closer to our own time, therapists and physicians have been researching music's ability to lower blood pressure, relieve chronic pain, and decrease the need for pain medication. Recently, researchers have also found that music may help reduce seizures.

About ten years ago, Dr. Gordon Shaw and colleagues at the University of California discovered that brain activity, when converted to sound output (as opposed to visual output such as an electroencephalogram), sounded like music. The sound resembled baroque, New Age, or Eastern music. If brain activity can sound like music, Dr. Shaw and his colleagues wondered, isn't it possible to work backwards and understand how music may influence the brain by activating similar neural patterns? They turned to Mozart for an answer because, they reasoned, the child prodigy began composing music at the age of four. Surely his brain would have been receptive to and actively engaged in this fundamental music-brain interchange.

They were right. In subsequent studies, the music of Mozart has been found to decrease epileptic activity in people experiencing seizures. John Hughes, M.D., a neurologist at the University of Illinois Medical Center in Chicago, conducted a study of thirty-six individuals, some of whom were in a coma or in *status epilepticus*. Twenty-nine of these patients showed a marked reduction in seizure intensity and frequency shortly after he began playing Mozart.[20] A more recent study of his of a child with Lennox-Gastaut syndrome showed that exposure to Mozart's Piano Sonata in D Major (opus K448) for ten minutes every hour during wakefulness produced fewer clinical seizures and fewer generalized bilateral spike and wave complexes over a twenty-four-hour period.[21]

What is it about Mozart, and specifically the Piano Sonata in D Major, K448, that is so powerful? According to Dr. Hughes, who analyzed hundreds of compositions by Mozart, Chopin, and fifty-five other composers, it may have to do with sequencing of musical patterns. He and a musicologist devised a scale that scores how often the music's loudness rises and falls in surges of ten seconds or longer. Mozart scored highest on this measure, while minimalist music by Phillip Glass and pop tunes scored lowest. Dr. Hughes believes that sequences that repeat every twenty or thirty seconds may trigger the strongest brain responses because many functions of the central nervous system, such as the onset of sleep and brain-wave patterns, also occur in thirty-second cycles. Naturally, there's been some controversy about these studies. But Dr. Hughes's research opens intriguing possibilities for using music to assist in seizure control.

Blocking Seizures

We tend to think of seizures as random, uncontrollable events. Yet, in a study of seventy-six adult and child patients attending an epilepsy clinic in England, Peter Fenwick, M.D., an epileptologist and psychiatrist, found that 36 percent of the patients stated that they could sometimes stop their seizures, without any training.[22] Surprisingly, between 25 and 33 percent were able to generate a seizure. (The children sometimes did it as revenge on their parents.) But it's also possible to learn to avert one.

To do this, you need to have an aura, or a forewarning absence seizure. If you experience an aura before a seizure, it's possible that you can do more than lie down quietly and wait for the storm to pass. By using certain mental or sensory techniques, you may be able to avert a seizure entirely—not every time, perhaps, but by averting the ones you can, you increase your sense of control.

It's estimated that about 70 percent of people with epilepsy have auras. I don't have auras, but I'm fascinated by them. One woman in my epilepsy support group described hers as a "bright white light in front of me for about a minute." Another person said he used to have a searching aura. "My mind would take over," he said, "and I'd think there were roaches or lice in my pocket and I'd keep looking there. Once, in a nightclub, I started going through some woman's purse. Now my aura is a knife piercing my back. It feels like a door opening and closing."

An aura is a way your body communicates with you to warn you of an impending seizure. This allows you to either find a safe place to lie down or to stop the seizure activity from spreading. To identify your aura (also called a *prodrome*), keep a diary for several months of activities, food and beverages, sleep, exercise, and feelings that precede each seizure. Try to locate any common factors. Ask friends and family if they notice any behavior—irritability, say, or facial expressions—before a seizure. (A friend of mine said she could always tell when her grandfather was about to have a seizure because his eyes would dart to the side.)

Once you recognize your aura, you can learn to block a seizure. People whose seizures have focal onsets sometimes say "no!" to themselves or try to switch their attention to something else at the beginning of the aura. Since mental imagery affects the neurochemistry of the brain, a person can effectively stop a seizure through meditation or visualization at an aura's onset. You can sometimes abort a seizure by focusing on your breathing. One researcher observed that children in a special school had fewer seizures when attending classes that were stimulating, such as art, and that patients in general had fewer seizures when their interest was held, such as when watching a movie or on vacation.

If a person's aura is a scent, another scent may block the seizure. Dr. Robert Efron described a woman whose seizures were preceded by an unpleasant odor. He gave his patient a vial of jasmine to sniff whenever she smelled this disagreeable odor, and that prevented the spread of the seizure discharge. Later, he taught her how to imagine the odor of jasmine and to thereby block her seizures. She was able to gradually stop medication.[23]

A tingling sensation or trembling is a common aura. When the tingling begins in a hand, arm, or leg, you can quickly apply a ligature or tourniquet just above the line where the sensations stop but in the direction where they are headed. This pressure seems to create a barrier in the region of the brain involved in control of that arm or leg. You can also use pinpricks above the line of tingles.

Touch is another sensation that can effectively block a seizure. Dr. Efron described a mother who tickled her child when she observed his aura, a turning of the head. Sometimes a gentle slapping can stop a seizure as well.

Epilepsy researchers have long suspected that too much synchrony among too many neurons may signal the onset of a seizure. Researchers Klaus Lehnertz and Christian E. Elger of the University of Bonn in Germany, using a complex mathematical system from chaos theory, have demonstrated that "a loss of complexity" due to coordinated nerve firing can be detectable in brain waves an average of eleven minutes before the start of a seizure.[24] They are currently testing whether patients whose seizures originate in the hippocampus—a region of the brain that deals with memory and learning—can avert seizures by conjuring specific memories or learning particular tasks. They also hope to develop an implantable monitor that could provide a warning of a seizure or automatically deliver electrical stimulation to prevent the seizure. However, the safety of putting electrodes on or in the region where seizures originate is in question.

For a comprehensive and detailed description of stopping seizures, read *Epilepsy: A New Approach*, by Adrienne Richard and Dr. Joel Reiter. Richard has taught workshops for people with epilepsy and has a great deal of experience in blocking seizures.

Who Needs Sleep?

At the end of the nineteenth century, Americans averaged about nine hours of sleep a night. Now we average about seven and a half hours. We seem to believe as a culture that needing sleep is a weakness;

however, sleep allows our bodies to carry out numerous critical bio-chemical activities. Sleep is necessary to help our brains deal with stresses and upsets of the day and to problem-solve through dream-ing. We all need a particular amount of sleep to "recharge."

Lack of sleep is a leading cause of seizures. This is especially true for people who have learned methods to deal with seizures, including conscious relaxation, dealing effectively with stress and emotional triggers, and other methods that require some conscious effort. People simply don't have the energy to employ these methods effectively when they are overtired.

Research has shown that lack of sleep changes the brain pat-terns of electrical activity.[25] Seizures arising from sleep deprivation may also be due to neurochemical or hormonal changes. It's possi-ble that the normal increase in protein synthesis that occurs during sleep may be hindered, and cellular repairs can't be made at the usual rate; this may render brain cells more vulnerable to seizure activity. (If you are tired, be sure to take precautions around heavy machinery.)

Most people with epilepsy experience seizures when awake, but some have seizures during sleep, and some have a mixture of both. It's not unusual for people who have seizures to also suffer from sleep disorders, such as sleepwalking, nocturnal enuresis (bedwetting), and night terrors. Nocturnal seizures are a possible cause of bedwetting and can occur during any sleep stage. Sleepwalking and night ter-rors may represent disorders in or arousal from slow-wave sleep, or deep sleep. Often, unrecognized depression, which may be related to medication, is at the root of sleep problems. Some medications (including Dilantin and Felbatol) can cause insomnia. If you or your child is having problems sleeping, consult your physician.

It's best to establish a routine of going to bed at the same time every night and preparing yourself with a relaxing activity, such as reading, writing in your journal, watching television, or taking a warm bath or shower. Do aerobic exercise regularly but not within four hours of bedtime. It may help to drink a cup of valerian tea before bed. Definitely avoid alcohol, sleeping pills, and tranquilizers. For mild insomnia, says nutritionist Gary Null, about 1,500 mg of calcium citrate and magnesium citrate before bedtime should be helpful. About 50 mg of vitamin B_6, along with 500 mg of inositol, also helps to promote sleep. Herbs such as ashen flower, skullcap, valerian root, and catnip may also be helpful.[26]

The deceptively simple act of breathing is a natural tool for stress management and seizure reduction. Dr. Weil has commented that "proper breathing nourishes the brain and central nervous system. If breathing is impaired, the natural movements of the brain and the membranes and the fluid covering it, are not adequate." Gay Hendricks, author of *Conscious Breathing*, says, "On a purely physiological level, if you learn how to breathe deeper and more powerfully, you actually grow more capillary space in your body."

We can reprogram our brains, grow more blood cells to transport more oxygen to the brain, and use our imaginations to deeply relax. We can change our bodies and behavior in numerous ways that improve our health and reduce seizures. Says Adrienne Richard, "We have and can exert much more control over our neurophysiological states than was once thought possible."[27]

CHAPTER II

Body Therapies

> *Listen to your body; it has the wisdom to know what is good for it.*
>
> —FROM "CHOICES," THE NEWSLETTER OF CITIZENS FOR ALTERNATIVE CARE

Touch can have powerful effects on humans. We know that babies who are not touched and held develop far more slowly than those who are. The idea that touch can heal is ancient; the first written records of massage, for example, date back three thousand years.

Whether a trained therapist manipulates muscles to make them more relaxed or to clear energy pathways, that gentle, therapeutic contact somehow activates energy systems in another person. Of course, even when a friend massages your aching feet, that feels wonderful, too. But does all this have actual health benefits for a person with epilepsy? The amount of rigorous scientific data to suggest the efficacy of therapies such as acupuncture, chiropractic manipulation, or various massage therapies is very limited. Still, the few studies that have been done, as well as case studies, indicate that many people have found these therapies to be beneficial, stirring interest among researchers. This chapter will discuss a number of body therapies that may be helpful.

Acupuncture

This ancient method of preventing and treating illness forms the basis for traditional Chinese medicine. In a healthy person, the Chinese believe, the *qi* flows unimpeded. *Qi* is the life force or vital energy that is involved in all bodily functions, from metabolism to emotions. When the flow or circulation is impeded, illness results. Therefore, the goal of acupuncture is to restore harmony (yin and yang) within the body. Acupuncture is not a self-help treatment; it must be performed by a licensed practitioner.

Physicians detect the pulse of only the heart in a patient's wrist, but acupuncturists can also feel pulses of the stomach, spleen, intestines, and liver. At the beginning of each treatment (which lasts about a half hour), an acupuncturist detects the flow of *qi* by feeling the patient's pulses, thus checking points that give information about how the body is working.

To balance energy, the acupuncturist inserts very fine, sterilized, stainless steel needles, little thicker than a hair, at key points along the body to access the twelve channels, or meridians, where *qi* flows through the body. (For a person with epilepsy, this would certainly include points that influence brain energy to increase the flow of blood to the head.) This process manipulates the energy flow, either increasing or decreasing the *qi* at various points in the body to help clear energy blockages. Because acupuncture treatments are aided by a person's lifestyle and diet, many acupuncturists make dietary recommendations and prescribe herbs to help ensure that the correction in energy flow lasts.

In the United States, much of the research on acupuncture has been done on dogs. In one study of five dogs, all had decreased numbers of seizures after being treated with acupuncture. Three continued to have fewer seizures with lower levels of anticonvulsants; the other two dogs also had a reduction in seizures while taking the same amount of medication, but they reverted back to their previous pattern five months after their last treatment.[1] Studies in China have shown acupuncture to be a safe, reliable way to reduce or lower seizure activity. One study, reported in *Epilepsia* magazine, indicated that treatment of epilepsy with a combination of herbs, acupuncture, and massage had the best results.[2]

There are several variations on acupuncture. These include:

- Acupressure, which involves massaging acupuncture points
- Ammatherapy, a form of Oriental massage therapy that focuses on the balance and movement of *qi* throughout the body
- Moxibustion, or heat treatments, in which a small container of burning herbs is placed inches away from the skin
- Shiatsu, a traditional Japanese healing art, wherein a practitioner may use fingers, elbows, knees, and feet to stimulate the flow of the patient's energy, break down energy blockages, and restore balance

A few people have found that acupuncture may stimulate seizures. This result may be because the acupuncturist isn't very skilled, or it's possible that like some treatments, you feel worse before you get better. Or perhaps it just doesn't work for some people.

Chiropractic Manipulation

Chiropractors specialize in diagnosing and treating mechanical disorders of joints, especially joints of the spine. The underlying principle is that misalignments in the vertebrae can interfere with the circulation of blood, lymph, and nerve activity to vital organs, causing a variety of illnesses. Chiropractors usually take x-rays when making a diagnosis; treatment involves brief, direct manipulations of the spine. (Since the spine is part of the nervous system, it makes sense that problems there could cause seizures.) Some chiropractors also use heat treatment and massage and offer recommendations regarding nutrition.

In a study reported by J. Alcantara, published in the *Journal of Manipulative and Physiological Therapeutics*, a chiropractor described treating a woman with low back pain who had had seizures since childhood. She had absence and tonic-clonic seizures, having a seizure approximately every three hours. After chiropractic adjustments to the subluxations at the cervical, thoracic, and lumbopelvic regions, the woman's low back pain improved and her seizure frequency decreased. At a follow-up a year and a half later, she said her seizures were less frequent, with periods between seizures as long as two months, and she no longer had back pain. The author concluded that the "results encourage further investigation of possible neurological sequelae, such as epileptic seizures, from spinal dysfunction identified as vertebral subluxation complexes by chiropractors and treated by specific spinal adjustments."[3] In another case, Dr. Lendon Smith recalls a boy experiencing seizures who received chiropractic adjustments for four months. Since the adjustments, he's been completely free of seizures. (He even tried out for the Philadelphia Eagles football team.)

Craniosacral Therapy

Most doctors are taught in medical school that the bones of the skull become fused together at the age of thirty-five or younger; after that, the bones are immobile. However, much research indicates that human skull bones aren't fused together until much later in life. This mobility underpins craniosacral therapy.

The word *craniosacral* can be broken into two parts: *cranio* refers to the cranium, or head, and *sacral* refers to the base of the spine and tailbone. Basically, the craniosacral system is composed of the brain and spinal cord (the central nervous system); the cerebrospinal fluid that bathes them; the surrounding membranes, or meninges, that enclose the brain, spinal cord, and cerebrospinal fluid; and the bones of the spine and skull that contain these membranes. Craniosacral therapy manipulates the bones of the skull to treat a range of conditions, including headache, spinal-cord injury, ear infections, epilepsy, and autism. Generally practiced by osteopaths, craniosacral therapy is used to evaluate and treat problems involving the brain and spinal cord, especially direct trauma to the head and spine.

Imbalances in the craniosacral system sometimes begin before birth. Inadequate prenatal nutrition can result in underdevelopment of the facial and jaw bones that may later impair harmonious functioning of the craniosacral system. Also, difficult deliveries can cause stresses to the growing cranial tissues. Many of these stresses to the newborn's craniosacral system are normally considered untreatable by conventional medicine or go unnoticed. However, should a person experience birth trauma, a bike accident, or a car accident that years later precipitates seizures, migraines, or headaches, craniosacral therapy can help take pressure off the central nervous system, lowering the stress load.

"When there is synchronous movement in the craniosacral system, the physiology of the central nervous system functions more efficiently and the nerve tissues in general are healthier," says Robert Norret, D.C., director of Stillpoint Health Center in Venice, California.

There are slightly different approaches to craniosacral therapy. In the sutural approach, a therapist manipulates the sutures (where the bones meet) to ease pressure and increase mobility of the cranial bones. The meningeal approach focuses primarily on manipulating the underlying membranes, or meninges, to dispel tension or restriction. The reflex approach focuses on relieving stress in the craniosacral system and in other parts of the body. By stimulating nerve endings in the scalp or between cranial sutures, this technique helps the nervous system to turn off stress signals.

A system of craniosacral therapy that combines the sacral, meningeal, and reflex approaches is the sacro-occipital technique (SOT). Also known as "craniopathy," SOT helps remove restrictions between the cranial bones and in the craniosacral system. This approach aims at improving structural stability and neurological functions.

A cranial therapist is trained to palpate, or feel with his or her hands, the integrated movement of the bones. The touch is extremely gentle and sensitive, but a therapist can diagnose the movement of the bones by locating critical points of restriction in the cranium. Practitioners may use massage, manipulation, or stretching, perhaps manipulating parts of a person's skull that were pushed out of place by a car accident, head trauma, or even from a difficult birth. A therapist may seem to be doing little more than pleasant touch, but he or she can assess a person's spine position, breathing, and how areas of the skull conform to that. Since therapy can take the pressure off the central nervous system, osteopaths believe this can help reduce the intensity and frequency of seizures. A therapist can also inadvertently promote a seizure by treating someone with epilepsy. Paul Dart, M.D., of Eugene, Oregon, who has treated several children whose seizures have become less frequent, says, "I have no way of identifying how a person will react beforehand."

Although craniosacral therapy has wide applicability, it has not been well researched. Therefore, information about its efficacy has been available mostly through case reports. One such report tells of a naturopathic doctor who helped a nine-year-old girl reduce her tonic-clonic seizures from one every three to four days to none. In addition to the craniosacral treatments, the naturopath helped the girl's parents make changes in their daughter's diet such as including supplements of flaxseed oil and eliminating wheat. Two years later, she remained seizure free but continued with occasional sessions of craniosacral treatments because she found the gentle massage very relaxing.[4] Viola Frymann, D.O., director of the Osteopathic Center for Children in San Diego, says she has treated many children, from infancy through adolescence. "Some children have ceased to have seizures and are free of anticonvulsant medications," she says. "Some children have been able to reduce medication but are not yet free from seizures." Often craniosacral therapy is combined with other treatments, such as homeopathy and nutrition.[5]

Massage

Massage is an Arabic word meaning "to stroke." That is precisely what massage therapists do: they stroke an individual's body with varying intensity and force to correct inadequacies in the musculature and nervous system. The tomb of Ankh-mahor, dating back to 2200 B.C., depicts an Egyptian priest giving a man a foot massage.

Therapeutic massage evinces reduced heart rate and lower blood pressure and causes the brain to release endorphins, the brain's natural opiate, which promote stress reduction and encourage the brain to make alpha brain waves. These effects can help decrease seizure frequency or eliminate seizures altogether. Massage—like reflexology, Rolfing, and shiatsu—treats the body as a whole rather than concentrating on physical conditions alone.

Reflexology

Reflexology is a system of diagnosis and treatment carried out by massaging the feet. Reflexologists believe the bottoms of your feet have points that correspond to every organ in your body and that the body is divided into ten energy zones that correspond to different areas of the feet. By massaging certain areas of the foot, it is possible to bring about a response in the corresponding tissues of the body. For example, points by the sole or heel correspond to the brain. Although no one knows how reflexology works, it is useful in a number of ailments and particularly useful in cases where the area of injury or problem cannot be touched or treated directly, such as in the brain.

Be sure to contact a reputable practitioner who has treated people with epilepsy and favors a gentle approach. According to the British Reflexology Association, overstimulation can trigger seizures.

Rolfing (Rolf Method of Structural Integration)

This system, a form of therapeutic massage, was developed over decades by Ida Rolf. Its applicability to epilepsy has not been researched. However, the goal of Rolfing is to allow the body to move naturally into good posture by eliminating the causes of skeletal misalignments and restoring the body's fascia (connective tissue that holds your body together, giving it shape) to a healthy state. Rolfing strives to release muscle tension, which increases the amount of available energy and eliminates energy losses caused by the strains and chronic muscle contractions in a misaligned, unbalanced body.

Usually, over ten sessions lasting about an hour each, a therapist works on a client, who lies on a padded table. The Rolfer applies pressure with fingers, hands, or elbows to release strains and distortions in fascial structures to restore the body to balance. In the past, critics of Rolfing complained that it was painful, but more modern techniques have addressed ways to alleviate the pain some people experienced.

Alexander Technique

Developed by F. Mathias Alexander, an Australian actor, this movement therapy strives to improve mental and physical well-being through changes in posture. Alexander suffered severe vocal difficulties and studied his own habits of movement to determine what might be causing these difficulties. He realized that he habitually tensed his neck muscles with the intake of each breath, which resulted in a distortion of the head-neck-spine relationship and a consequent interference with natural coordination. He promoted a system of movement reeducation to increase bodily awareness, ease of movement, and clarity of thinking. The technique aims to allow the body to have perfect balance and poise with minimum muscular and mental tension.

Lessons in the Alexander Technique are available from professionals at dance schools and community colleges. Once you have learned the movements, you can perform the exercises on your own.

Aromatherapy/Flower Essences

Our sense of smell can be a powerful ally. Knowledge of how odor can be used to stimulate, relax, and heal has been passed down through the centuries and was refined in the early twentieth century. Essential oils, obtained from plants, roots, leaves, flowers, and fruits, have been shown to have powerful psychological effects. Research has shown that certain oils, when inhaled, have the power to relax or stimulate.

Bach Flower Remedies were invented and used in the 1930s by Dr. Edward Bach, an English homeopathic physician. The remedies are derived from combining wildflowers and pure stream water, which Dr. Bach believed would provide subtle energy that is effective in treating ailments, taking into consideration an individual's mood and emotional outlook.

Aromatherapy hasn't been very well researched in the United States, though it has been researched extensively in Europe, where it is widely practiced. One study at the Seizure Clinic at Birmingham University in England used aromatherapy on fifty patients who were unresponsive to seizure medication. Reportedly, sixteen patients became seizure free after one year; for seventeen others, the number of seizures was reduced by half.[6]

Aromatherapy can be a safe, effective self-care treatment, but follow these guidelines:

- Use the purest oils available from reputable suppliers.
- Avoid contact with the eyes.
- Keep essential oils out of the reach of children.
- Always close your eyes when inhaling essential oils.

Essential oils are highly concentrated. When placed on the skin, they are nearly always diluted with a carrier oil (sunflower, safflower, or almond, for example) or an emulsified oil and water lotion. The dilution needed is different for the treatment of each ailment. When making a dilution, add the required drops of oil to the carrier oil or lotion and shake well.

We tend to think of epilepsy as being merely a brain difficulty. But when we have a seizure, our whole body experiences it, so it is only appropriate that we should learn to use, quite literally, our senses or a combination of senses to prevent seizures. Our senses are an unexplored resource with great potential for self-healing.

How Neurotoxins Affect Our Nervous System

Prolonged exposure to toxins and metabolic abnormalities can lead to structural damage and recurrent epileptic seizures.

—JEROME ENGEL, M.D., FROM "SOME ENVIRONMENTAL EXPOSURES ASSOCIATED WITH SEIZURES" BY LOUISE KOSTA

A growing number of researchers are warning of the dangers of neurotoxic chemicals in our environment. Conventional farming methods rely on massive use of synthetic pesticides, herbicides, and fertilizers, a number of which are known neurotoxins. These chemicals are ingested when people eat food sprayed with these harmful chemicals. In addition, we eat these chemicals when we eat meat from animals that have fed on plants sprayed with pesticides. Hundreds of millions of pounds of pesticides are sprayed on crops each year. Yet, less than half of seventy thousand approved pesticides are tested for neurotoxicity.

Pesticides, heavy metals (such as mercury, aluminum, lead), and neurotoxins present in common household and garden products can adversely affect our nervous system. Hundreds of different toxins stored in our fat can pass through the blood-brain barrier and the placenta. Children and fetuses are particularly at risk, due to their low weight and developing nervous systems. Since a pesticide's purpose is to kill living organisms, what potential effect might it have on humans, especially humans prone to seizures?

Pesticides

The generic term *pesticides* also refers to insecticides (insect killers), herbicides (weed killers), and fungicides (mold killers) sprayed on crops, lawns, school grounds, and other places where plants abound. Agricultural and industrial use of pesticides has grown considerably, but most of these chemicals have not been adequately studied for their safety for general health and should be avoided. Much of the scientific research that has been done indicates that some of the ingredients in widely used commercial pesticides contribute to an array of health problems.

Pesticides that have been associated with convulsions include aldicarb, chlordane, chlorthion 2, and 4-D (DDE, DDT, demetion, and dieldrin).[1] In addition, permethrin inhibits a nervous system receptor, the GABA receptor, producing excitability and convulsions. The most toxic pesticides, organophosphate pesticides (OPs), are chemically related to nerve gases developed by the Nazis during World War II. Products such as the widely used insecticide malathion, the chlorinated hydrocarbon insecticides lindane and dieldrin, and the formamidine insecticides amitraz and chlordimeform are routinely used on farms and gardens. OPs, of which there are about forty-five, attack the nervous system; these neurotoxins inhibit an enzyme that is essential for normal transmission of nerve impulses from one nerve to another.

Some OPs are approved for more than one use. Chlorpyrifos, for example, another widely used chemical, is known under the trade names Dursban and Lorsban. Dursban had been approved by the Environmental Protection Agency (EPA) for uses ranging from termite control to flea collars. The EPA approved the same insecticide (under the name of Lorsban) for use on more than a hundred crops, including corn and apples. Concerned by the thousands of reported cases of poisonings that occur yearly within homes, schools, and parks, the EPA announced in spring 2000 that it would phase out Dursban for nonagricultural uses and curtail the application of Lorsban on some crops that are frequently eaten by children, including apples.

While many health advocates are pleased that the EPA is enforcing a law passed by Congress in 1996 that requires the EPA to impose much tougher restrictions on the use of pesticides found to pose a special risk to children, they are disappointed that products containing Dursban may remain on store shelves until December 2001 and can still be used in some areas, such as golf courses and houses under construction. They're also dismayed that the EPA did not pursue broader restrictions on Lorsban for agricultural uses. "When the EPA identifies hazards it should stop their use," said Jay Feldman, executive director of the National Coalition Against the Misuse of Pesticides.

The use of known neurotoxins where children may come in contact with them is of particular concern because children's nervous, metabolic, and immune systems are still developing, so they are more susceptible than adults to the harmful effects of some pesticides. Recent laboratory studies on animals have shown that exposure to pesticides while the nervous system is developing can cause long-lasting, possibly permanent effects on the nervous system.

"Some pesticides—the pyrethroids—interfere with biochemical interactions in the brain and cause seizures," says Mary Gilbert, Ph.D., based on her research on the effects of pesticides.[2] In Dr. Gilbert's study the animals developed seizures following low-level injections of several kinds of pesticides. Once this degree of sensitization to seizures has occurred, other seizures occur more readily. Apparently the seizure threshold is lowered. One such pyrethroid insecticide, cypermethrin, is used to kill insects on cotton and lettuce, and to kill cockroaches, fleas, and termites in houses and other buildings. Permethrin, in the synthetic pyrethroid family, is used to kill insects in agriculture, for home pest control, forestry, and head lice.

Then there is an herbicide used to control weeds on farms and lawns called glufosinate, which chemically resembles glutamine, a molecule used to transmit nerve impulses in the brain. Following exposure to glufosinate, laboratory animals experienced convulsions, disequilibrium, and diarrhea.[3]

Kindling

Exposure to neurotoxins (and all toxic substances) can affect the central nervous system in two ways: either an acute toxic reaction may occur or a chronic low-level exposure, called kindling, may cause seizures, along with other physical problems. Neurotoxicity tends to be cumulative and permanent, as damaged brain cells do not regenerate.[4] There are no nerve endings in the brain to sense pain and warn of cell injury.

Researchers have found that seizures occurred when either chemical or electrical currents were repeatedly applied to animals' brains, even if each irritant was incapable of causing a seizure by itself. Similarly, kindling occurs when a repeated irritation causes changes in behavior and in the brain's electrical activity. According to neurologist Clause Wasterlain, kindling is "the progressive buildup, in response to intermittent low-intensity electrical or chemical stimulation of certain brain sites, of cellular discharges, culminating in full-fledged seizures."[5] Exposure over a prolonged period is more insidious and harder to detect.

Until recently, pesticide regulations in the United States considered pesticides individually, without regard for the total number of different pesticides a person might consume on a single fruit or vegetable. A 1993 report by the National Research Council recommended that the regulatory process be changed so that it could account for simultaneous exposure to multiple pesticides that affect our health the same way.

It's best to buy organic produce (food that has been certified as having been grown without any pesticides) from a farmers market, food co-op, or health-food store; or grow food in your own garden. According to a Rutgers University study, a significant difference exists between organic and commercially grown produce. When tested in a laboratory, the mineral content of the organically grown produce proved to be as much as 75 percent richer. There was also a significant increase in the amount of trace minerals, including iron, manganese, boron, copper, and cobalt. Currently, there are no federal standards for organic produce. Each state certifies its own organic growers, so standards may vary.

Your grocery store may be able to provide you with information regarding fruits and vegetables grown using few or no pesticides. These foods are often grown using integrated pest management (IPM), but as with organic produce, there are no national standards on these farming methods.

If you must buy produce that has been sprayed, health professionals make the following recommendations:

- Wash and scrub all fresh fruits and vegetables thoroughly under running water. This will help remove bacteria and traces of chemicals from the surface of produce and dirt from crevices. However, not all pesticide residues can be removed by washing.
- Peel fruits and vegetables when possible to reduce dirt, bacteria, and pesticide residue. Also, trim fat from meat and skin from poultry because some pesticides collect in fat.
- Vary foods. Eating a variety of foods will give you a better mix of nutrients and reduce your likelihood of exposure to a single pesticide.

Pesticides in Baby Food

A study conducted by the Environmental Working Group (EWG) found sixteen pesticide residues, some of which are possible carcinogens and several of which are toxic to the nervous system, in the eight most commonly eaten baby foods. All were produced by the three major baby-food manufacturers, Gerber, Heinz, and Beech-Nut. In general, EWG's analysis found that canned fruits contained more pesticides than the vegetables. About a quarter of the squash samples tested contained DDE, the breakdown product of the organochlorine insecticide DDT, or dieldrin, another organochlorine whose agricultural use was banned in the United States in the 1970s.[6] It is very disturbing to know that nearly thirty years later we are still feeding residues of these dangerous chemicals to our babies. (After being pressured by consumers, Gerber has announced that it is dropping suppliers who use genetically engineered corn and soybean products, and it is trying to switch to only organic ingredients in its products.)

In addition, scientists from the Environmental and Occupational Health Services Institute of Rutgers University tested plastic and felt toys found in rooms sprayed with the insecticide Dursban. Even two weeks after spraying, the researchers were still finding chlorpyrifos on the toys. They recommend that toys be put away during, and for many days after, spraying.[7]

Heavy Metals

Heavy metals, such as lead, mercury, cadmium, and aluminum, can induce seizures by disrupting neural function once they are absorbed into the brain.[8] Pesticides and heavy metals also affect the nervous system. One well-known example is lead poisoning. Lead is carried through the body in the bloodstream. Even though the blood tends to eliminate its burden of lead, the amount carried into the brain remains, and in high concentrations it can harm the nervous system and cause seizures.

Symptoms of lead poisoning among children include seizures, trembling of facial muscles, and ringing in the ears. Adults may experience disequilibrium, awkwardness, seizures, and unsteadiness in feet and hands. If you think that you or your child has lead poisoning, see your doctor immediately. The most effective treatment is chelation therapy, in which certain chemicals that bind with the heavy metals are injected into the body and "escort" the heavy metals out, mainly through urination.

Aluminum and mercury should also be avoided. High levels of mercury can cause birth defects and brain damage in infants. Products routinely used around the house that may contain aluminum include painkillers, deodorants, and antacids; many foods contain aluminum, including some commercial brands of table salt and some flours. (Aluminum cookware, once suspected as a source of aluminum absorbed by the body, seems to have been exonerated.)

Health-food stores carry substitutes, such as sea salt and aluminum-free baking soda.

Aluminum hasn't been directly implicated in seizures, but research has shown that it has the potential to damage the brain or nervous system. It appears that nerve cells are more vulnerable to heavy metals, such as aluminum, when magnesium levels in the brain are low. Magnesium plays a vital role in protecting brain cells from the harmful effects of neurotoxins. Research has shown that aluminum inhibits certain enzymes involved in producing acetylcholine, a neurotransmitter that plays an important role in memory function. Aluminum is being studied for its possible implications in Alzheimer's disease.

Tuna and other freshwater fish and seafood, say many experts, can contain dangerous levels of mercury. The fish are often contaminated by emissions from coal-fired plants, incinerators, and other industrial facilities that end up in the water, where mercury turns into its organic form, methylmercury, and accumulates in fish tissue. Methylmercury is a neurotoxin that affects the nervous system and brain development.

Mercury is a well-known neurotoxic agent that has been linked with various types of mental disturbance (which is why some dentists no longer use mercury amalgams for dental fillings). According to Jackie Savitz, executive director of Coast Alliance, a coalition of three hundred environmental groups across the United States, pregnant women represent the number one risk group for mercury contamination through consumption because mercury can cross the placenta.

Heavy metal toxicity should be ruled out as a possible cause in all seizures. A hair mineral analysis provides the best screening method for the detection of heavy metals. More sensitive tests can be used if necessary.

Genetically Engineered Foods

Genetic engineering, or biotechnology, has made its way into our agricultural system and onto our dinner tables. Genetic engineering is a laboratory technique used by scientists to change the DNA of living organisms. The DNA is the blueprint for the individuality of an organism, which relies on the information stored in its DNA for the management of every biochemical process. Segments of DNA are called genes, and scientists learned how to build customized DNA using genes. They also learned about vectors, strands of DNA like viruses, which can infect a cell and insert themselves into its DNA. With such knowledge, scientists can build vectors, incorporating genes of their own choosing, and use the new vectors to insert these genes into the DNA of living organisms.[9] But they haven't inquired about whether such activity is a safe thing to do.

Although such foods, referred to as genetically modified organisms (GMOs), present a threat to human health and the environment, there has been limited public debate or media scrutiny, particularly in the United States. The biotech industry, working with the government, has introduced these foods quietly, unlabeled, and mixed in with other foods. Interestingly, there is already staunch consumer opposition to genetically engineered foods in Europe, where GMOs are called "Frankenfoods."

The September 1999 issue of *Consumer Reports* stated: "Genetically engineered foods are already on supermarket shelves—in baby formulas, tortilla chips, drink mixes, taco shells, veggie burgers, muffin mix—and even in fast food fare." People who suffer from allergies could be exposed to food they react to without knowing it. A few years ago, researchers showed that a Brazil nut gene spliced into soybeans induced allergies in people sensitive to the nuts.[10]

In June of 1999, lawyer Steven Druker of the Alliance for Bio-Integrity charged that the FDA disregarded the warnings of its own scientists about the unique risks of gene-spliced foods.[11] According to professor Mae Wan-Ho of the U.K. Open University, "The insertion of foreign genes into the host genome has long been known to have many harmful and fatal effects, including cancer of the organism." Professor Richard Lacey, M.D., a microbiologist, argues against introducing genetically engineered foods because of the "essentially unlimited health risks" that they pose. Peter Will, Ph.D., a biologist at Auckland University in New Zealand, says that cellular proteins replicated in other species can give rise to infectious neurological disease.

By transferring genes across species barriers that have existed for eons, scientists risk changing the blueprint of each organism's biological processes. Genetically engineered foods reproduce themselves and can never be recalled from the environment; nor can they be kept apart from their wild and nonaltered relatives. One field testing of genetically altered potatoes indicated that, over distances of 1,100 meters, 72 percent of the nonmodified potatoes contained the transmuted gene.

Currently, labeling of GMOs is not required despite the fact that, worldwide, the vast majority of people want GMOs to be properly labeled, and efforts are under way by the biotech industry to prevent nonaltered foods from being labeled as "biotech free." GMO crops are mixed with nonaltered crops, so it is virtually impossible for the average consumer to avoid eating genetically altered foods. To best avoid the possible toxic side effects of these foods, buy organic produce as much as possible, avoid processed foods, eat rennetless cheese, and avoid dairy products that are not organic.

Certified organic foods are presumed safe from genetic engineering. However, pollen from a GMO crop miles away can infiltrate organically grown crops. And seed can get mixed in the bins in processing plants. In addition, processed foods may contain up to 5 percent of nonorganic ingredients, and these could be genetically altered. For example, organic ice cream might contain organic milk and organic cream but also contain lecithin from genetically altered soybeans. At the very least, insist that genetically engineered foods be labeled, and let your grocery store know that, for the sake of your family's health, you won't buy genetically engineered foods.

Unquestionably, we live in a very polluted world and much of our food supply is unsafe. Buying organic produce or growing our own, avoiding toxic household and garden products, and pressuring our public officials are major ways we can minimize our exposure to these toxins. We need to demand basic information about pesticide use: which pesticides are being sprayed on the food we and our children eat or on the soccer fields, school grounds, and lawns where our children play; how much is being used; and what, if any, side effects exist. We need to know where and how our food is grown. Ultimately, the only way to avoid the contamination of our environment by harmful chemicals is to stop their use.

PART IV

Age, Gender, and Epilepsy

CHAPTER 13

Children and Epilepsy

It is virtually never appropriate to accept that your child must be significantly limited by his seizures. You have to believe that your child can fulfill his own potential.

—JOHN FREEMAN, M.D., AUTHOR OF *Seizures and Epilepsy in Childhood*

An estimated 350,000 children in the United States have epilepsy. Approximately one-third of these children will outgrow their seizures; however, the experience can be traumatic for all children. Educators, doctors, and psychologists agree that children with epilepsy shouldn't be made to feel left out or singled out. Part of this is physical—being able to participate in sports like other kids. And part of this is academic and social—doing well in school, joining extracurricular activities, making friends. Ensuring that children aren't left out may require extra patience and consideration on the part of teachers and parents to supply the encouragement and love the children need and emphasize their skills and achievements.

Neonatal Seizures

Not all seizures in infants are due to epilepsy. Seizures in newborns can have many causes, such as problems with brain development before birth, lack of oxygen during or following birth, a head injury, nutritional deficiencies (especially lack of vitamin B_6), or the after-effects of severe brain infections such as meningitis or encephalitis. In addition, being exposed in the womb or through breast-feeding to excitotoxins consumed by the mother may trigger a seizure. Seizures in children can also be caused by high fevers, infections, head injury, or lead poisoning. It's estimated that one out of every twenty-five children will have at least one febrile seizure. These usually occur in children between the ages of six months and five years. Although they're certainly frightening to parents, most febrile seizures are benign, not causing brain damage. Between 95 and 98 percent of children who have them do not develop epilepsy. However, although the risk factor is small, certain children who have febrile seizures face an increasing risk of developing epilepsy. Epileptic seizures in newborns (called neonatal seizures) are often difficult to recognize because they may not appear to be much different from normal infant behavior. Parents often feel guilty for not recognizing a seizure from the beginning, but they can be subtle and brief, and even nurses and doctors may have difficulty recognizing them. For this reason, neonatal seizures can go undiagnosed until they occur frequently or dramatically.

To make a diagnosis, a physician will usually ask for a full account of pregnancy, labor, and delivery, as well as what the infant did before the convulsions and other circumstances. Because newborns' brain development is incomplete, interpreting their EEGs can be difficult. Many EEG tracings that would be considered abnormal in older children are actually normal for infants, so diagnosis might include urine and blood tests and CT or MRI scans.

Distinguishing Seizures from Nonseizures

While seizures can begin at any time of life, 50 percent of all cases of epilepsy begin before the age of twenty-five; many start in early childhood.[1] But just because a baby jerks her arms and legs sometimes doesn't mean she's having infantile spasms. Just because a child stares into space doesn't mean he's having an absence seizure. Children frequently stare at nothing, daydreaming. Children who are daydreaming will respond if you call their name; children having an absence seizure usually won't. On the other hand, if a child is hard to wake up in the morning, has sore muscles, and has wet the bed, this could possibly indicate a seizure has occurred during the night. A child may induce a nonepileptic seizure by hyperventilating, or overbreathing. If such symptoms persist or if you notice behavior such as limb twitching, eye rolling, or body rocking, consult a physician.

Helping Kids with Brain Damage

Some children develop epileptic seizures from birth trauma, strokes, brain hemorrhage, or exposure to environmental toxins. But if their bodies are receiving the nutrition they require, it is possible to raise the seizure threshold.

Following are several studies involving children and the effects of vitamin supplementation on seizures:

- Twenty-four children whose seizures were not controlled by medication were divided into two groups. Those in the experimental group were given 400 IU of vitamin E daily in addition to their anticonvulsant medication. The children in the control group were given placebos. After three months, six of the twelve children receiving vitamin E reduced their seizures 90 to 100 percent. Four children experienced a reduction rate of 60 to 90 percent. Two were noncompliant. When the children on placebo were given vitamin E, seizure frequency in all of them was reportedly reduced 70 to 100 percent.[2]

- At the Great Ormond Street Hospital for Sick Children, which is located in England, a study conducted on children found that shortly after specific food allergies had been identified and the allergen(s) removed, migraine headaches and epilepsy disappeared in seventy-eight out of eighty-eight children.[3]

- Thirty epileptic children with tonic-clonic or absence seizures were given 450 mg of magnesium daily, and their anticonvulsant medications were discontinued. Twenty-nine reportedly showed significant improvements in seizure control. One thirteen-year-old child who had a ten-year history of uncontrollable seizures had shown signs of retardation. After receiving magnesium, his seizures stopped and his mental capacity improved.[4]

- Many anticonvulsants can cause liver problems, weight gain, rashes, even behavioral difficulties. But a number of studies also indicate that children taking anticonvulsants are at risk for bone loss and delay in bone development. Some researchers recommend that vitamin D supplements be given to children who have taken medications for two years or more. In one study, bone loss was evident in severely handicapped children with epilepsy who were institutionalized, getting little exercise. When given vitamin D supplementation, at 4,000 IU daily for six months, their bone mineral content improved.

Brain Growth

Scientists have recently discovered that a child's brain undergoes dramatic anatomical changes between the ages of three and fifteen. Brain scans show that between these ages, the brain grows quickly in some areas—mirroring a child's physical growth spurts—but shrinks in others.

Previously, researchers had assumed that major neurological growth took place in the womb or very early in childhood and that the overall structure of the brain changed very little, if at all, after the age of five or six. But in new brain-scan studies, brain images indicated that the growth process continues into adolescence. The amount of gray matter (bulk neurons that are not yet permanently "wired" into neural circuits) in some areas of the brain can nearly double within as little as a year, followed by a correspondingly drastic loss of tissue as unneeded cells are purged and the brain continues to organize itself.

Neuroscientists have long known that a two-stage process of growth and attrition is typical of brain development from fetal development through early childhood. The brain produces gray matter. These cells then begin to arrange themselves into patterns, depending on which connections are reinforced by an individual child's mental or physical activity. The least-used cells and pathways die out in a phenomenon scientists call pruning, wherein white matter (primarily fibers interconnecting nerve cells) forms to firm up the most robust connections.[5]

In a study by researchers from the University of California at Los Angeles (UCLA) and McGill University in Canada, scientists conducted successive three-dimensional brain scans of several normal children over intervals as short as two weeks and as long as four years. Researchers focused on size and shape changes in a complex nerve-fiber network called the corpus callosum, which connects the brain's right and left hemispheres. Scientists consider it a reliable indicator of the level of activity in different parts of the brain. These results indicated that from age three to six, the most rapid growth in the brain takes place in the frontal lobes, which are involved in planning and organizing new actions and in maintaining attention to tasks.[6] But during the period from six to puberty (which occurs around age eleven in girls and age twelve in boys), the growth of gray matter shifts to the temporal and parietal lobes, which play a major role in language skills and spatial relations.

As children grow older, this growth appears to move in a sort of wave from the front of the brain to the rear. "We were quite surprised," says Jay N. Giedd, a child psychiatrist with the National Institute of Mental Health in Bethesda, Maryland, "to see this unexpected increase in gray matter in the front part of the brain right before puberty." This unexpected increase in gray matter, researchers noted, was followed by a loss in the frontal lobes from the midteens through the midtwenties. (The frontal lobes control the higher functions of the human mind, such as memory, mood, cognition, and consciousness. They are also essential for inhibitory impulses, regulating emotion, and organizing behaviors.)

Dr. Giedd believes that the rule for brain structure appears to be "use it or lose it." What is thought to happen next is that if a person is doing sports, academics, or music, those are the abilities that are going to be "hard-wired" as the circuits mature. The teenage years are a critical time to optimize the brain. In other words, teenagers actually have a say in how their brains develop.

Indeed, although it is true that a child's brain grows very fast until about age three, research has found that the brain is highly adaptable through much of our lives. While the life experiences of babies and toddlers affect the organizations of their brains, scientists still don't know which of those changes are permanent or long-lasting.

How might this information help children with epilepsy? It might help to explain why some children apparently outgrow their seizures. For example, in benign childhood epilepsy, also known as Rolandic epilepsy, seizures almost always disappear after adolescence. If the area of the brain from which a seizure begins is purged, seizures might change or disappear. (Sometimes they manifest in others ways, such as migraine headaches.) Also, in terms of the neuronal pruning, research is beginning to show that if something happens to interrupt that process, such as a serious accident or trauma to the frontal lobes, the results can be devastating. A child who has sustained brain injury, for example, may seem to make a physical recovery, but once he or she reaches adolescence, cognitive and behavioral problems may start to show. It might also shed some light on why and how some children's seizure patterns change.

Teenagers with Epilepsy Have Special Needs

For any teenager, coping with emerging adulthood is a major life challenge. A chronic disability such as epilepsy magnifies the problems of adolescence. And the consequences of seizures at this time can be more severe than in childhood. Ironically, it's a time when teens often feel invincible.

At a time when deviations from peer groups assume great importance and self-consciousness increases, having seizures can be disastrous for an adolescent's self-esteem and sense of identity. If he or she knows others with epilepsy or other disabilities, that can be a great opportunity for friendship. Driving, the use of alcohol and recreational drugs, sexual relationships, and the possibility of pregnancy are issues that teens must consider, and when the teen has epilepsy, these issues gain a whole new spectrum of challenges. While no one wants to rob adolescents of exhilarating experiences or opportunities, they are exposed to more risks. In general, common sense prevails, with a need for supervision to regulate adequate sleep, not smoking, responsible sports participation, and so on. Driving depends on laws, which vary from state to state. Openly discussing epilepsy at home can help form a foundation for good habits that will serve adolescents well into adulthood.

As a child matures into adolescence, his or her seizures may end. For example, Rosie had absence seizures as a child and took Tegretol for three years. As a teenager she became seizure free. But she began having migraine headaches. As nutritionist Jerri Spalding Fredin has observed in her article "New Hope for People with Epilepsy":

> How many epilepsy researchers have studied people who have "outgrown" their seizures? Did they "outgrow" their seizures, or did they "grow into" some other kind of sensitized reaction? One mother told me her child had "outgrown" his seizures but was having migraine headaches, which he had not previously had; and migraines can be triggered by food sensitivities.[7]

Nutrition

For those teenagers whose seizures have not ended, new coping strategies must be found. For example, one epilepsy center advocates consultation with a neurologist, pediatric neurologist, and a nurse specializing in epilepsy. In these meetings, the focus is on the needs and independence of the teenager, with parents taking a back seat.

A nutritionist should probably be added to this team. As children mature, their nutritional needs often change; nutritionists can evaluate their needs and discuss nutrition and vitamin supplements with them. Teens, whose diets can no longer be supervised as closely, are notorious for eating fast food and junk food. Such a diet isn't great for any adolescent, but for one prone to seizures, it can be quite harmful and could possibly bring on seizures, particularly if the teens are hypoglycemic. (Perhaps we should warn them that junk food causes pimples!)

Medication

Compliance with medical treatment is of particular concern in this age-group. For teenagers, there is intense peer pressure to conform, to be seen as "normal," and their pills are a reminder that they're not like everybody else. Additionally, side effects of medication may be magnified; whereas, for example, gum growth or hyperplasia from taking Dilantin was once tolerable, now it's not. So teens may decide on their own to take less medication or to take it only intermittently. Having friends who have seizures or other disabilities is one of the best ways to reinforce healthy habits, as well as deepen their friendships, making them feel more like they fit in.

Sex and Sexuality

It's a fact of life that most teenagers are giddy with sexual matters—although sex is usually an uncomfortable topic between adults and adolescents. While parents feel teenagers aren't ready for intimate sexual relationships, their kids may not feel the same way. As I said, many teenagers feel invincible. But if they engage in sexual intercourse, it can complicate their lives in ways they never anticipated.

For instance, although using contraceptives is responsible behavior, oral contraceptives may fail. A Johns Hopkins study found that women taking certain anticonvulsant drugs (such as Dilantin and Tegretol) experience a failure rate of oral contraceptives of 6 percent or more a year. Women should be advised of this—by their physician or pharmacist—and either find alternate sources of birth control or abstain from sex. They should also be told that, according to various studies, the possibility of birth defects for women who are taking anticonvulsants is 4 to 8 percent, double the risk for nonepileptic women. There is evidence that taking daily folic acid supplements reduces this risk. Since it's estimated that about 30 percent of teenage pregnancies are unplanned, a number of doctors recommend that those having sexual intercourse take 5 mg of folic acid daily.[8]

There are few studies of males who have epilepsy, and those few that do exist indicate that males taking anticonvulsants experience lower serum levels and lowered sex drive (hyposexuality). These side effects can have a deep impact on an adolescent male's psychological state and his behavior, particularly if the anticonvulsants interfere with hormones that affect male sex characteristics, such as body hair, voice change, and so on. This area certainly requires further research.

On a more sober note, child sexual abuse, particularly incest by alcoholic fathers and father-surrogates, has been implicated in absence and complex partial seizures. Meir Gross, M.D., who studied a number of such cases, recommends that "For every adolescent who is presented to the clinician because of hysterical seizures [without organic cause], a detailed history should be taken, including information about the family dynamics, with particular attention to the possibility of incest."[9] Such physical abuse, in boys as well as girls, calls for medical and psychological intervention.

Parents As Caregivers

If you've ever flown in an airplane, you're familiar with the safety message that flight attendants give before takeoff. After telling us how to buckle the safety belts and how to use the seat cushion as a flotation device, they tell us what to do if the cabin loses pressure: "An oxygen mask will drop down from the bulkhead. If you are traveling with a small child or someone who needs assistance, put your mask on first and then assist the other person." That advice is a good metaphor for caregivers: you can't help someone else if you are gasping for air. But that is often what caregivers, especially parents, seem to be trying to do. You can't give and give and give without renewing your energy. We fill our cars up with fuel when the tank is empty; we need to do the same for ourselves.

Seizures, behavior problems, getting help, emotional stress, and developmental and medical problems were most frequently cited by a group of parents as the most difficult problems in caring for children with epilepsy. Molly Eastman, who conducted the study for the Minnesota Epilepsy Group, urged more help for parents in coping with these issues.

Seizures

It is possible for parents to gain a sense of control, even if the seizures themselves are not controlled. Developing a plan for how to handle the disruption a seizure causes, becoming more flexible, and not overscheduling family activities help to reduce frustration. Counseling, either family or individual therapy, can also help resolve difficulties. Support groups can be an invaluable means of support and sharing problem-solving tips. After all, nobody but another parent of a child with seizures can possibly understand what you are experiencing. To locate a parents support network near you, contact the Epilepsy Foundation at (800) EFA-1000.

It's important to learn all you can about a child's illness and physical condition, as well as treatment options. Also, says James Murray, R.N., the "importance to inform children about their medical condition cannot be overstressed. Children often have secret fears and feelings of guilt surrounding their illness."[10]

Behavior Problems

A number of professionals have identified parents' "benevolent overreaction," which includes overprotection of a child with a handicap, overindulgence, and permissiveness—or, as some would say, "spoiling." This benevolent overreaction doesn't allow parents to see through the illness and realize their child's potential for independence. Instead, parents frequently become trapped in a cycle of indulgence and overprotection, both in times of frequent seizures and in relatively seizure-free periods.

Unfortunately, such behavior can be detrimental to the child's emotional welfare, leading to low self-esteem and lack of initiative. In some cases, parents perform actions for the child that the child is capable of doing, such as answering for the child or assisting with dressing, toileting, or feeding. Giving children age-appropriate responsibilities and allowing them to take part in health-care decisions when appropriate are important. Applying the same rules to them as to their siblings and peers in regard to discipline, household chores and activities, and attending school is necessary to promote growth and maturity. Deprivation of such experiences can result in emotional, social, and intellectual handicaps worse than the epilepsy itself.[11]

Sometimes, children who are overprotected by parents actually exhibit hostile behavior toward them—cursing, slapping, and spitting at parents—behavior that parents often overlook. Perhaps such hostile reactions should be taken by the parents as an indication that the child is craving independence and responsibility.

Getting Help

In a survey conducted in 1995 by the National Family Caregivers Association, 65 percent of the respondents said they didn't get any assistance from family or friends.[12] There is also a lack of available support services for children, and parents are overwhelmed by having to locate services within the health-care system. Many times, parents experience feelings of entrapment, despair, frustration, and anger. One mother, whose daughter had intractable seizures as well as numerous cognitive and physical handicaps, felt suicidal. Another mother, distraught by the distance family members have kept, admits she may have facilitated this by acting so "strong" at the beginning and taking on all of the caregiving responsibilities herself. Now, family members feel free not to help out. They may feel that if they were to offer help it would only be turned down anyway or perhaps they're afraid of stepping on toes because it was always made clear that she didn't need help.

But it's crucial that parents ask for help. Family members and friends may need concrete suggestions. For example, Martha, a single mother of an eight-year-old boy with Down's syndrome, called a family meeting and told everyone how difficult it was caring for her son. She made it clear that she needed assistance and couldn't shoulder the responsibilities by herself anymore. Then Martha distributed a list of all the ways people could help out and asked them to tell her which activity they would be willing to take on. Her strategy worked. Now she has two committed weekly helpers. When asked why he wasn't helping earlier, Martha's brother said, "She didn't ask."

Emotional Stress

The emotional stress of caring for a loved one is immense. As one mother said, "We are five years into this hellish roller-coaster ride known as intractable epilepsy. In the early days of my son's seizures, I prayed that this hideous nightmare would just go away altogether. When that didn't happen, I came to accept the epilepsy and just prayed that we could get the seizures under control. When that didn't happen, I learned to just take it one day at a time. But I still have not stopped praying. He is my son. I love him. And he is my hero."[12]

The normal grief, guilt, and anger felt by many parents with chronically ill children can lead to more stress in the family dynamics. Even if we know that our child's illness and bureaucratic hurdles are not our fault, we nevertheless feel we are somehow at fault. Jaime Lyn Bauer, an actress whose son has epilepsy, has written:

> One parent, usually the father, is in denial. Denial brings about isolation of the other parent and the child with epilepsy. That child is often rejected and blamed by the parent in denial in an attempt by the parent to distance himself or herself from the problem. This places tremendous pressure on the marriage relationship and, ultimately, on the entire family.[14]

To help relieve some of the emotional burden, health-care professionals stress the importance of finding time for yourself. Even if it's only a few minutes a day, time spent writing in a journal, doing yoga or meditation, or spending time in the garden will replenish your energies. It will also keep your frustration, depression, and exhaustion levels from building.

Caregivers also need to participate in activities away from the child, though we often feel too guilty to do so. Yet if we don't take care of ourselves, if we deplete our resources, we'll have nothing left to give. This can lead to depression, insomnia, and intense arguments. In one study at a comprehensive epilepsy center, parents were encouraged to participate in activities for themselves. Some parents who did said it was the first time in several years that they had been separated from their child.

Developmental and Medical Problems

It's estimated that up to 15 percent of children below the age of eighteen have some chronic illness. In addition to learning as much as possible about a child's illness, parents must focus on what the child *can* do. If parents overindulge a child with epilepsy, the child is deprived of new learning experiences, discipline, and structure. The child remains dependent on the parents and parents may react to this behavior with frustration, perhaps even resentment; these emotions are transmitted to the child, who may react by withdrawing, feeling increased stress, or being irritable.

Encourage your children to ask you and their physician questions. Not talking about the illness gives children the impression that you are ashamed of their medical condition and makes them feel ashamed of having seizures. There is still a cultural stigma surrounding epilepsy, one that children with asthma or diabetes don't have to battle, so it is important to prepare children with epilepsy with the appropriate knowledge and self-esteem.

When a Parent Has Epilepsy

Parents with epilepsy often wonder when and how to explain their seizures to their children. Some parents whose seizures are controlled never tell their children; however, this may only reinforce the fear and anxiety surrounding seizures. One teenager I spoke to said he first saw his mother have a seizure when he was fifteen. "At first," he said, "I though she was fooling around. Then I realized it was no joke."

Parents may believe that their children are too young to understand seizures. However, children understand much more than we think they do, and talking about it when a child is two or three probably isn't too early. (One researcher mentioned an eighteen-month-old boy who was so aware of his father's seizures that he could imitate them perfectly.)[15] A parent can explain what is happening to Mommy or Daddy in simple, concrete terms, such as, "When Mommy falls or spaces out, she's having a seizure. She'll be OK in a minute."

It's very important to let children know that something is happening and to reassure them that they are safe. Nobody is in danger. When a seizure occurs, Mom isn't dying. As the children get a little older, a parent may even tell them what to do in case of a seizure: call a grown-up; make sure Mom isn't near anything hot, like an iron or a stove. Seizures can be described in a little more detail to a school-aged child. Nancy Stalland, a psychologist, and Patricia Osborne Shafer, a neuroepilepsy nurse specialist, make these suggestions:

- Show children photographs of the brain and body.
- Encourage children to draw what they think happens during a seizure.
- Encourage children to talk about how they feel during a seizure.
- Older children might speak to the parent's health-care practitioner for practical information.
- Support groups for children of parents with epilepsy may be available.[16]

These things not only help influence how children cope with a parent's seizures but also make epilepsy more real and, therefore, less frightening. Failure to explain seizures may increase children's fear and anxiety, making it more likely that they will blame themselves for the seizures or make up bizarre fantasies to explain them.[17]

Writing an instruction list of simple steps for children to take if their parent is having a seizure and posting the list in an accessible area (on the refrigerator or a bulletin board) will help the children stay calm during the seizure. Having occasional seizure "drills" lets everyone know how to help.

If a parent's seizures are too severe or frequent to allow them to carry out daily responsibilities, it's not uncommon for children to take on extra responsibilities, such as cooking or shopping. The parent may become overly dependent on the child, inadvertently reversing caregiver roles. Children may also try to protect their parent from emotional or stressful situations, concealing their own problems for fear of upsetting the parent. Undoubtedly, this can increase stress in children.

Too often, family caregiving decisions are made in the heat of a crisis and long-term implications of these decisions aren't thought out. When possible, families need to project ahead, envisioning where each member will be three or five years from now, advises Dr. John Rolland, associate professor of psychiatry and codirector of the Center for Family Health at the University of Chicago. That way, he says, the burdens of caregiving can be spread around and one person won't end up making all the sacrifices. It also helps put decisions in perspective because the goal is family stability, and with that perspective it's possible to realize that the entire family is affected by epilepsy.

CHAPTER 14 ————————————————

Women and Epilepsy

Epilepsy complicates every aspect of a woman's life. The woman with epilepsy faces medical, legal, social, educational, and economic challenges. Few chronic illnesses carry the impact of seizures.

—Elizabeth Borda, former director of the
Epilepsy Foundation of America's Women
and Epilepsy Initiative

About the same number of women as men have epilepsy. But having epilepsy can affect women far more significantly. Women face special concerns related to menstruation, birth control, pregnancy, birth defects, and menopause. Studies have shown that as a group, we experience:

- Lower marriage rates
- Reduced fertility
- Sexual dysfunction
- Fewer children
- A mortality rate twice that of men with epilepsy and twice as high among nonwhite women with epilepsy compared to white women

Hormones and Seizures

Hormones are chemical substances that control biological processes
such as muscle growth, heart rate, and menstrual cycle. Steroid hormones include the three major sex hormone groups: estrogens,
androgens, and progesterones. All of these are present in men and
women but in different amounts. Research has shown a connection
between hormones and seizures, though that connection is just
beginning to be understood. The female hormones estrogen and
progesterone act on certain brain cells, particularly those in the temporal lobe. Estrogen is proconvulsant, while progesterone has a
seizure-protective effect.

There are an estimated 800,000 American women of childbearing age with epilepsy. According to Martha Morrell, M.D.,
chairperson of the Epilepsy Foundation, more than one-third of
women with epilepsy experience disorders of sexual dysfunction.[1]
Unfortunately, seizures, or the fear of having seizures, can restrict
opportunities for forming and maintaining intimate relationships.

Fertility

Anticonvulsants can alter hormone levels and reduce fertility. A
study done by the Institute of Neurology in England of more than
2 million people with epilepsy discovered that women in the general
population had a 33 percent higher fertility rate than those with
epilepsy. This corresponds to Dr. Morrell's findings that fertility
rates in women with epilepsy are one-third those of nonepileptic siblings. It's also possible that these women don't want to have children
for fear their child will inherit the epilepsy.

It's not uncommon for seizures to begin at puberty, intensify-
ing what for most young women is one of the most dramatic, chal-

lenging, frustrating times in their lives. Seizures that begin in childhood may improve at menarche, or they could worsen. Janet Mims, in an article in the *Journal of Neuroscience Nursing*, writes:

> While resources are directed at the adult female with epilepsy, there is minimal information available for and about adolescent females with epilepsy. Adolescence is a time of change in body image, hormonal balance, and social expectations. Issues of sexuality and socialization are difficult to address in children without chronic illness. . . . There may be additional concerns regarding issues of sexuality in an adolescent with epilepsy.

She also believes that health practitioners should make extra efforts to discuss nutrition and vitamin supplements with their young patients during puberty and menarche.[2]

Menstruation

Approximately 30 percent of women with epilepsy report catamenial (menstrual-related) seizures, with their seizures more likely to occur before menstruation. Hormones play the largest role. Before a woman begins her period, her estrogen level rises. The brain is more irritable and more likely to seize when estrogen levels are high. On the other hand, progesterone, with its seizure-protective effect, is lowered. If a woman is taking medication to treat epilepsy, the hormones may alter the efficacy of the drug.

In addition, starting a few days before the menstrual period, women's bodies temporarily eliminate the medications faster than usual. Water accumulates in the body to compensate for the fact that it is about to lose a lot of fluids. The brain is the most pressure-sensitive organ in the body, so it feels water retention the most acutely. One physician describes it as "literally, a kind of pressing down." This pressure can cause premenstrual seizures. Some researchers also think that just before menstruation there is a drop in calcium, magnesium, and B_6 levels, nutrients that help raise the seizure threshold. Some evidence also indicates that the ovaries may swell, affecting the spinal cord.

To help relieve bodily tension around the time of menstruation, practice relaxation exercises and deep breathing. Vitamin B_6 is a natural diuretic, so eating foods rich in this vitamin will help reduce water retention. Cutting down on fluid intake may be helpful as well as avoiding sugar. According to Dr. Morrell, women with epilepsy have a higher frequency of anovulatory menstrual cycles (missing periods) and abnormal menstrual cycle length than nonepileptic women. Fluctuations in reproductive hormones occur in those women who are and those who are not treated with anticonvulsants, but medication can interfere with those functions.

Taking progesterone may help women who have catamenial seizures. In one study, twenty-five women who experienced complex partial or secondary generalized seizures of temporal origin around the time of their period were given doses of progesterone three times a day during certain days of their cycle for three months. Eighteen of the twenty-five women reported fewer seizures during that time frame.[3]

Sexual Dysfunction

More than one-third of women with epilepsy experience disorders of sexual arousal. According to Dr. Morrell, epileptic discharges can disrupt the function of brain structures mediating sexual behavior, such as the limbic cortex, and can disturb hypothalamic and pituitary hormone release. Anticonvulsant medications can affect sexual behavior through alterations in hormone metabolism and direct effects on cortical function.[4]

Another factor in sexual dysfunction is the feeling that having a disability like epilepsy is not sexy or desirable. We tend to feel ashamed of our bodies, which we feel can betray us at any moment, and this perhaps contributes to feelings of inadequacy. A study that evaluated self-reported sexual function in women with epilepsy found a high incidence of dyspareunia (pain during intercourse), vaginismus (painful vaginal spasms during intercourse), and lack of vaginal lubrication. However, these same women reported no problems in sexual desire or experience, so their problems may be related to fears of intercourse. Having orgasms, losing control, or hyperventilating may be thought to trigger a seizure. (Notably, it is rare for people to have a seizure during sex.)

Moisturizing and lubricating products can facilitate smooth-muscle relaxation and vasodilation. Practicing deep diaphragmatic breathing can stimulate sexual energy. If problems persist, personal counseling or couples therapy may be of value. (Having any chronic illness can be unwieldy. For example, in a study comparing epileptic and diabetic women, 29 percent of the women with epilepsy reported sexual difficulties, while 28 percent of the diabetic women reported sexual problems.)[5]

Birth Control

Women who have epilepsy often find it difficult to speak to their doctors about birth control and other matters of sexuality. For example, a few months after a woman in my epilepsy support group underwent brain surgery, she was seeing her neurologist for a checkup. When he prescribed new medication for her, she asked him if it would interfere with her birth control pills. He callously replied, "Why would you want to take birth control pills?" as though incredulous that she might want to enjoy a sex life. It's also disturbing that in a telephone survey of 345 women conducted by the Epilepsy Foundation, 46 percent of the women said their concerns were not taken seriously by their doctors.

All available birth control methods can be used by women who have epilepsy. These include:

- Barriers: diaphragms, spermicidal vaginal creams, intrauterine devices (IUDs), and condoms
- Timing: the rhythm method, in which intercourse is avoided during a woman's ovulation period, and withdrawal by the man prior to ejaculation (these are the least reliable methods of birth control)
- Hormonal: birth control pills, hormone implants, and hormone injections

There is no evidence suggesting that taking birth control pills will adversely affect epilepsy. There are, however, complex interactions between the hormones estrogen and progesterone in birth control pills and anticonvulsants, which can influence the metabolism of the pill and thereby reduce its effectiveness. Some medications, such as carbamazepine (Tegretol), phenytoin (Dilantin), phenobarbital, primidone (Mysoline), and topiramate (Topamax), have been found to lower concentrations of estrogen by as much as 40 or 50 percent.

These medications, often called liver-enzyme-inducing drugs, increase the breakdown of contraceptive hormones in the body, making them less effective. Medications such as valproate (Depakote) and felbamate (Felbatol) do not increase breakdown of hormones and may even increase hormonal levels. Gabapentin (Neurontin) and

lamotrigine (Lamictal) reportedly do not interfere with the effectiveness of hormonal birth control. (One survey found that 85 percent of gynecologists and neurologists the researchers contacted
didn't know that anticonvulsants can make hormonal birth control
less effective.)

A Johns Hopkins study found that some women with epilepsy
developed unplanned, perhaps unwanted, pregnancies because their
medication interfered with birth control pills. They may experience
a failure of oral contraceptives of 6 percent or more a year. Using
contraceptive pills with higher doses of estrogen may help, but even
this is no guarantee of 100 percent efficacy. For women taking one
of the anticonvulsants that speed up the breakdown of hormones in
birth control, doctors advise considering barrier methods of contra-
ception. If you have decided you definitely don't want to have
children, women can undergo a tubal ligation or men can get a
vasectomy.

Pregnancy

In the past, women with epilepsy were discouraged from having
children. In some cases, they were sterilized against their will. But
epilepsy is no longer demonized. Well over 90 percent of women
with epilepsy who give birth have safe deliveries with normal,
healthy children. Still, women with epilepsy tend to have more pregnancy complications, such as premature labor and vaginal bleeding.
About 25 to 30 percent of women with epilepsy have more frequent
seizures during pregnancy, while a similar number find that seizures
are less frequent.

Studies indicate that the fetus is most vulnerable to anticonvulsant medications during the first trimester (which is when the
spinal cord develops). Risk of major birth defects, such as cleft lip

or palate, for infants born to women without epilepsy is 2 to 3 percent. However, according to Dr. Morrell, in women with epilepsy who use anticonvulsants, the risk rises to 4 to 6 percent. She adds that there may be minor birth defects in up to 20 percent of babies born to mothers with epilepsy, which may be caused by the complex interactions among drugs, genetics, nutritional deficiencies, and other factors. Because of these risks, many women think about lowering medication, but this can also be risky because a seizure during pregnancy could potentially harm the fetus (the potential for harm is greatest in the case of a tonic-clonic seizure because the developing baby's oxygen supply is cut off). The risks and benefits of lowering or forgoing medication during part or all of a pregnancy should be thoroughly discussed with your doctor.

Nutrition

Ideally, women ought to speak to their doctors about pregnancy before or soon after becoming pregnant. It's recommended that women taking medication who plan to become pregnant take a supplement of folic acid, about 4 or 5 mg per day, before conception. Studies have shown that folic acid deficiency is a worldwide problem, and for all women, folic acid supplementation lowers the risk of neural tube defects, such as spina bifida. Researcher Janet Mims recommends that all females of childbearing potential receive folic acid to decrease the possibility of birth defects as the result of anticonvulsant therapy. A lack of B_6 and magnesium is closely associated with convulsions, which may be prevented by an adequate supply of these nutrients in the diet.

The most important time for such supplementation, studies show, is the first four weeks of pregnancy, before women know they're pregnant. Eating foods rich in folic acid, such as dark green leafy vegetables, orange juice, and liver, is recommended; whole grains, nuts, and eggs have lower amounts. Supplementing with B$_6$ has been found to be extremely important for the healthy development of a baby's nervous system.

Yukio Tanaka, M.D., of St. Mary's Hospital in Montreal, Canada, has demonstrated a link between manganese deficiency and convulsions in humans. He also believes that pregnant women whose diet is deficient in manganese have a higher chance of giving birth to epileptic children than women who receive adequate manganese.[6] Dorothy Klimis-Tavantzis, Ph.D., an expert on manganese and author of *Manganese in Health and Disease*, recommends a daily 5 mg manganese intake for women and teenagers. A higher intake might be necessary for pregnant women. Supplementing the diet with vitamin K one month before delivery has been shown to reduce the risk of hemorrhage. For your specific nutritional needs, consulting a nutritionist may be very helpful.

Jay Holder, M.D., Ph.D., recommends chiropractic adjustments during pregnancy. He believes they can improve chances of a better delivery, less back pain, and a healthier child and lessen chances of a miscarriage. And, as mentioned in Chapter 4, excitotoxins such as aspartame and MSG can penetrate the placenta, so these should be avoided. Environmental toxins should also be avoided.

Seizures

Pregnancy raises additional concerns about seizures. During pregnancy, one-quarter to one-third of women report an increase in seizure frequency, despite sustained use of medication. Difficulties during labor include premature labor and a failure to progress, possibly caused by anticonvulsants. Women with epilepsy are twice as likely to have cesarean sections. But most women with epilepsy have normal deliveries, and only 1 to 2 percent will experience a tonic-clonic seizure during labor.

After the baby is born, different concerns for seizures arise. Being a new mother usually entails lack of sleep, and sleep deprivation can be a seizure trigger. Working out routines with family members who can feed the infant at night is essential so the mother can get as much rest as possible. Breast-feeding, yet another concern for new moms, is generally considered safe.

Research shows that only about 3 out of 100 offspring of mothers with epilepsy will develop the disorder. (That risk increases if the child's father has epilepsy, too.) Still, even though research shows that over 90 percent of women with epilepsy give birth to healthy children, many women continue to worry that their child will experience developmental delays or learning disabilities. And what if a physician advises a woman with epilepsy not to have a baby? "If that occurs," says neurologist Mark Yerby, "get a second opinion. If a physician says this simply due to a woman's having epilepsy, it's probably not appropriate."

Managing Menopause

"Menopause," says naturopath Liz Dickey, "is not a disease. It's a natural life event." As such, it should be treated with lifestyle and nutritional practices designed to mitigate any menopausal symptoms, such as hot flashes and nocturnal sweating, and to avoid seizures. Hot flashes, for example, can be eased with exercise, vitamins E and C, and by reducing consumption of meat, alcohol, sugar, and refined carbohydrates.[7] Eating more soy and flaxseed is helpful, as both contain natural estrogens that help balance the body's estrogen system. Because synthetic chemicals used in pesticides can upset the body's internal estrogen system, many naturopaths recommend avoiding meat and processed foods.

Many women have found alleviation of specific menopause symptoms by taking herbs such as black cohosh and the Chinese herb dong quai. Sometimes referred to as the female ginseng, dong quai has been used for thousands of years to treat menstrual problems. Chinese researchers have also found that it helps increase energy. (If you suffer from diarrhea or bloating, check with your health practitioner before using dong quai.) Black cohosh has been studied extensively in Germany and has been found to be effective in easing hot flashes and insomnia, as well as anxiety, depression, and nervousness associated with menopause.[8] Since anticonvulsants can cause bone loss, it's important to exercise regularly and provide your body with adequate amounts of calcium and vitamins A and D, which have been shown to slow the rate of bone loss. It's probably useful to have your bone density measured. A woman with a hip density one standard deviation (SD) below the mean for her age is seven times more likely to have a hip fracture than a woman with normal bone mass.[9]

Every woman experiences menopause a little differently. The limited research that has addressed the effects of menopause on seizures has found no consistent pattern in worsening or lessening of seizures. Little information is known regarding changes in seizures at menopause or with postmenopausal hormone replacement therapy. The average age of menopause is fifty-one, but it can occur any time from the midforties to the late fifties. Women with certain seizure disorders, such as post-traumatic or temporal lobe epilepsy, may experience early menopause.[10] One woman in her late forties, who had been taking Tegretol for fifteen years, went into menopause ten years earlier than any other woman in her family. "I've had fewer seizures since menopause, but I've had hot flashes for eight years," she says. "I'm producing no estrogen; my ovaries aren't functioning. I'm like a woman with a hysterectomy." She also has problems with cystitis and wishes that more research focused on women. "Research on Tegretol and the endocrine system," she says, "has so far been limited to males."

What's a Woman to Do?

There are no easy answers. Each woman needs to find what nutritional and lifestyle program works best for her. There are, however, a few simple things all women can do to ensure better health.

- Women taking anticonvulsants need to learn what the risks are and what their lowest optimal dose is. Since studies have shown that anticonvulsants can interfere with the body's absorption of vitamin D, calcium, and folic acid, lifetime supplementation may be necessary to ensure an adequate supply of these elements. Anyone expecting a baby needs to speak to her physician regarding the added risk of antiepileptic drugs (AEDs).
- Water retention, which is part of premenstrual syndrome, may be helped by cutting down on liquids and sugar and consuming extra calcium, magnesium, and B_6, which is a natural diuretic. Nancy Nina, R.N., suggests taking an herbal diuretic before menstruation.
- Regarding lack of sexual desire, there doesn't seem to be a female equivalent to Viagra. But in a recent column Ann Landers wrote: "Many people, both men and women, who wish to enhance their sexual performance, are now taking herbal products. They are less expensive than prescription drugs and have fewer side effects, and the results have apparently been very satisfactory." She adds that herbal products are not regulated by the Food and Drug Administration, so results may vary. Since

herbs may interact with any medication you are taking, even aspirin, check with your health practitioner.

More researchers are beginning to acknowledge women's needs. The Epilepsy Foundation has established the Women and Epilepsy Initiative (WEI), with research and educational programs aimed at women with epilepsy, the public, and providers of women's health care. Women who become pregnant while taking an anticonvulsant can enroll with the Antiepileptic Drug Pregnancy Registry. This pregnancy registry has been established by an independent scientific advisory group and financed by five pharmaceutical companies manufacturing anticonvulsant medications. Although one may question how independent a scientific group will be when it's financed by pharmaceutical companies, at least the companies are beginning to recognize that women are looking for more natural ways to keep themselves, and their babies, healthy and seizure free.

Men and Epilepsy

The cure is attitude.

—Steve Fishman, author of *Bomb in the Brain*

Little research has been done regarding how epilepsy specifically affects men. While the physical difficulties women face due to seizures and anticonvulsant medications can be scientifically verified, the difficulties men with epilepsy face are not so clear. They appear to be more psychological in nature. In our culture, males are expected to be in control, to be invulnerable to physical infirmities, and, as adults, to face heavy social pressures to protect and support their families, all while remaining sexually vital. Seizures challenge these notions. Men tend to have more problems with alcoholism than women, and several studies show a link between epilepsy and alcohol abuse. One study concludes that alcohol abuse is an important, though often undetected, cause of seizures.

Behind all the statistics, I think of the men I know who have epilepsy. All have had to rein in their careers. About half have married; none have children. I think of Stephen, whose fiancee confided to me that he'd had a seizure during lovemaking. Then there's Jason, whose aunt told him that when his mother found out she was pregnant, she didn't want him. She persuaded a gynecologist to inject certain chemicals into her womb to bring about an abortion. His mother denies this, but he suspects that it might explain why he began having seizures a few months after he was born. He doesn't know for sure and that's hard for him to live with. And Noah, whose medication makes it difficult for him to have erections. "But my wife is very loving," he says, "and we're both very creative."

Sexual Dysfunction

Men with epilepsy frequently complain of sexual dysfunction, especially impotence and loss of libido. A number of studies have estimated that reduced potency and hyposexuality (lowered sexual interest) occur in 38 to 71 percent of men with epilepsy.[1] The sources of these symptoms include medication and psychosocial and hormonal causes.

As with women, many of men's problems with epilepsy are closely related to hormonal disturbances. The few studies that have been done on men with epilepsy have found that androgen deficiency is very common. Androgens are responsible for activities of the male sex organs and development of male sex characteristics (such as facial hair). Androgen deficiency may also contribute to reproductive and sexual dysfunction and possibly increase seizure frequency. Research on epileptic women's health issues has established that many women are more vulnerable to seizures around the time of menstruation. But little research has been done regarding men's hormone cycles, if they do occur, to determine if there are times when they are more prone to seizures.

Sexual dysfunction is probably a complex interplay of semen

levels, desire, anticonvulsant drug levels, sex hormones, genetics, and mood. One study reported, "There appears to be a significant rate of sexual dysfunction, especially among males with epilepsy and with complex partial seizures in particular. This information is usually not volunteered by the individual, even though it is a significant source of worry and concern."[2]

Fertility

Most of the few studies of men with epilepsy have examined fertility and sex hormones. One of the most consistent findings is that, like women, men with epilepsy experience lower fertility rates. Men with epilepsy also report problems in achieving and sustaining erections and ejaculation, for which anticonvulsants may be partly responsible. (Such difficulties may respond to medications that facilitate smooth-muscle relaxation and vasodilation.)

Some studies have found lower semen levels among men with epilepsy. Anticonvulsants may reduce fertility through inhibition of sperm motility. One study found that seizures may have an effect on the male reproductive system and that phenytoin (Dilantin) may have a slight additional influence.[3] Several studies in England have identified alterations in the level of sex hormones, noting a decrease in levels of free testosterone, which underlies the disorder in sexual function. The researchers were concerned about the social and psychological consequences. (I'd be remiss if I didn't mention a British study that found that men who ate organic foods produced 43 percent more sperm than those who did not.[4])

Hyposexuality

One study found that hyposexuality was particularly significant among men with epilepsy, particularly those with complex partial seizures. Researchers have cited other risks in connection with this disorder—specifically, that there is a known relationship between sexual function and a person's psychiatric status in general and level of depression in particular. Another study of men with epilepsy found that just 8 percent of the men reported sexual dysfunction; in a similar study done with men who have diabetes, 44 percent of the men reported sexual difficulties. The researchers note that most of the men had their seizures under control and were very accepting of their illness. They concluded that epilepsy doesn't necessarily increase the risk of sexual dysfunction in males (or females).[5]

Career

Men are not raised to be dependent. For all the New Age Male rhetoric, our culture still expects boys to become invincible and prosperous. And men are expected to hide their emotions. These are unrealistic expectations that nearly all men grapple with. However, men with epilepsy come up against them in cruel ways that they often have a hard time acknowledging.

It has been estimated that 50 percent of people with epilepsy are underemployed or unemployed. But there is very little research on men with epilepsy and employment. As for anecdotal evidence, I personally know of a man who got fired from his job after having a seizure, though he later sued the company and got his job back. Another man also had a seizure at work and was fired. He worked for a railroad company and, unfortunately, his union didn't support his efforts to win back his job. He sued the railroad company, and five years later he got his job back.

Often, employment issues are much more subtle than someone getting fired. For example, an architect whose seizures were caused by a benign tumor in his left temporal lobe had a very stressful job as lead architect for a large housing project. He had a number of seizures during that project, one at work. He quit that job and began practicing architecture on his own. He feels that it's difficult to obtain work from local firms because they've heard about his seizures and would prefer not to hire him. (For more information on how to balance work and epilepsy, see Chapter 18.)

Other Risks

Like women, men taking anticonvulsant medication may experience loss of bone density. While older women often lose bone density due to the gradual loss of estrogen that accompanies menopause and may experience osteoporosis, or thinning of bone density, a University of Washington study found that 180 men ranging from twenty-two to forty-five years of age who took anticonvulsants had up to four times the risk of fracturing their hips than men not taking the drugs.[7] Since men are usually physically stronger than women, their seizures can be worse, too. One man, whose seizures occur during sleep, said, "One time I tore my shoulders out of their sockets. Another time I threw my back out." Another man said he had a seizure in the bathroom so intense he moved the toilet from its foundation.

Often, adolescent boys and men deny their epilepsy by not following medical regimens. A nurse told me about several men she knew who didn't always take medication prescribed for them. She said, "It's like saying, 'It's not that bad. Maybe if I stop taking medications or seeking alternatives, the seizures will go away on their own.'" The mother of a twenty-one-year-old boy who developed seizures when he was eighteen remarked, "Sometimes Ian self-medicates, altering his dosages, and that has sometimes brought on a seizure. He acts like he just wants the epilepsy to go away."

In general, men have a greater fear than women of exposing their vulnerabilities and have great difficulty in discussing their problems. They are much less likely to seek therapy. (Men have a hard enough time asking for directions; asking for medical help must be excruciating!) This inability to seek help or to discuss their difficulties may be why nearly twice as many epileptic men than women commit suicide.

Discussing any fears with a partner can go a long way toward relieving anxiety and bringing couples closer together. Professional counseling and support groups are excellent ways men can explore their fears, frustration, and despair. It's also an opportunity to share what they've learned about dealing with seizures in creative and satisfying ways, thus transforming their expectations of themselves.

Until the 1970s there wasn't any research focusing on women and epilepsy. Now that more research is being done, studies regarding men and the ways that they perceive epilepsy, how it limits their opportunities, and how it affects their psychological well-being must be included. When more men allow themselves to talk about these issues, that will be a huge first step.

CHAPTER 16

Epilepsy and the Elderly

More important than the battle against death and disease,
I have come to believe, is the battle against despair.

—A FIRST-YEAR MEDICAL RESIDENT

Persons aged sixty-five and older are in the fastest-growing age-group in the United States. They're also the fastest-growing group of people developing epilepsy.

The incidence of epileptic seizures rises dramatically after the age of sixty. Known as late-onset epilepsy, it is associated with more risk factors than at any other age. These risks include cerebrovascular disease, dementia, infection, trauma, and alcoholism. Older people with epilepsy are at risk for developing fractures from accidents and drug toxicity, as well. With the projected increase in average lifespan, epilepsy is becoming an important health-care concern.

Diagnosis

According to researchers, about 70 percent of older epileptic patients have partial seizures. However, it's harder to diagnose older people than any other age-group. Physicians must distinguish epileptic seizures from other cerebral, cardiovascular, or metabolic diseases that may show similar symptoms. While an aura, tongue biting, and incontinence during an episode can be indicative of epilepsy, memory loss that lasts for a few minutes to hours can appear to be a seizure but rarely is. Correct diagnosis and classification of seizures requires an accurate patient history, clinical observations, and EEG recordings; unfortunately, the EEGs of elderly people are somewhat difficult to read. And obtaining a reliable history of epileptic seizures from an older patient living alone may be very difficult.

According to researchers, the most common identifiable cause of late-onset epilepsy is a previous stroke; head injury, Alzheimer's disease, and brain tumors are also major causes. There are a multitude of causes of brain damage resulting in dementia. For example, ongoing bouts of severe hypoglycemia can cause accumulated brain damage that may look like ministrokes. Some of the medications often used to treat medical disorders such as high blood pressure and heart problems can depress brain function, which is especially harmful in elderly people. The elderly are more prone to head injury and therefore are more likely to get post-traumatic seizures.

There is also evidence that many older people with declining intellectual function often have suffered from "silent strokes." Strokes occur when a brain artery is blocked, thereby depriving that part of the brain of its blood supply. If the blocked vessel is a major artery, a serious stroke occurs. But if the blocked artery is small, it may go unnoticed. Over a long time, several of these strokes may occur until the accumulated damage finally destroys enough brain cells to cause brain malfunctioning. By the time some people have reached their middle to late sixties, they may have suffered these strokes, unaware that anything has happened. This can cause rapid deterioration in health and quality of life.

(Incidentally, although there is no research proving that aspartame causes brain tumors in humans, it is curious that from 1973, the year aspartame was approved by the FDA, to 1990, the occurrence of brain tumors in people over the age of 65 has increased 67 percent.[1])

Complications

Anxiety and depression have been reported in many older people with epilepsy. In one study, more than 37 percent of the elderly people studied showed such symptoms. Slowness and thinking difficulties have also been related to epilepsy. Irritability was another symptom frequently found among older epileptic patients. Interestingly, children and the elderly are most susceptible to depression from taking phenobarbital.

Older people, especially women, are at risk for bone loss and osteoporosis. Vitamin D supplementation helps slow bone loss, especially for those who don't get adequate sunlight or exercise, such as those in nursing homes. Antiepileptic medications may exacerbate this problem by adversely affecting bone metabolism and increasing the risk of falls related to drug toxicity. Physicians can evaluate a person's bone metabolism through measurement of bone density and other tests.

Seizures themselves may also be a risk. Although a seizure usually lasts only a minute or two, the contraction of all major muscle groups places considerable stress on the cardiovascular system. This is generally tolerated by younger people but may cause problems in the elderly, such as increased risk of hemorrhage in the brain.

Overmedication

No segment of the population is as overmedicated as the elderly. In our youth-obsessed culture, we do not honor our elderly as elders. A recent radio ad for a "natural" antiaging cream identifying old age as a "treatable disease" typifies this attitude. Since when did a natural process of the body become pathological?

If medication is prescribed to prevent seizures, lower doses may be needed by seniors because of their slower metabolism.[2] Toxic levels of certain anticonvulsants such as phenytoin (Dilantin), phenobarbital, and carbamazepine (Tegretol) can cause neurologic difficulties, including problems with coordination and cognition, which may increase the risk of falling. Furthermore, anticonvulsants can interfere with other medications (such as glaucoma eye drops, high blood pressure medication, and laxatives) that interact with each other and with antiepileptic drugs, possibly contributing to further neurological side effects. Drug interactions may also result in a lowering of therapeutic drug levels or development of toxic side effects. The elderly may experience more side effects from drugs and are at greater risk for harmful drug interactions due to multiple drug therapy.

One nursing home survey revealed that residents were being given phenytoin (Dilantin) in doses similar to those given to younger adults, so they were probably being overdosed. According to Ilo Leppik, M.D., phenobarbital must be used cautiously in the elderly due to its propensity to cause sedation, depression, and mental slowness, which can be confused with the onset of dementia.

In another survey of nursing homes, 10 percent of the residents were taking at least one anticonvulsant. The use of anticonvulsants in the general elderly population still living in their own homes is likely to be less than those in nursing homes. Sadly, a major goal of some nursing homes is to keep patients sedated.

A further problem in nursing homes and retirement communities is that many patients receive medication such as phenytoin or phenobarbital for unknown and undocumented reasons. This occurs most often when the medical staff changes frequently, the initial records are lost, and when family members don't know why medication was prescribed in the first place.[3] For this reason, it's important to ask health professionals, for yourself or a loved one, "Why are these medications necessary?"

Nutrition

Nutritional needs of older people, especially in institutions, are much neglected. The food in some nursing homes is similar to hospital food, which is infamous for its lack of nutrition. And many older people living at home are on fixed incomes and may not be able to afford nutrititious meals. Indeed, some older people will skip meals to pay for prescription medication. In addition, decreased mobility as an elderly person makes preparing meals much more difficult.

Certain precautions can help minimize risks of developing epilepsy after age sixty: control high blood pressure, a risk factor in strokes; eat a healthy diet low in fat and salt; and avoid foods that contain excitotoxins, particularly MSG, hydrolyzed vegetable protein, and aspartame—these have been implicated in neurological damage, including seizures, Alzheimer's disease, brain tumors, and Parkinson's disease and, when eaten over decades, destroy brain cells. The accumulative damage is seen as we age.

Another good precaution is to take vitamin supplements, including:

- **Magnesium.** Supplementation of magnesium is helpful because it has been shown to raise the seizure threshold. Several studies have indicated that the elderly often do not eat vegetables, such as broccoli and spinach, or other foods that are high in magnesium. Recent nutritional studies indicate that up to 75 percent of adults in the United States have a significant magnesium deficiency. This deficiency increases with age and makes the brain more vulnerable to glutamate and aspartate.[4]

- **Vitamin B$_{12}$.** Low brain levels of this vitamin have been found to cause severe intellectual deterioration. Since B$_{12}$ deficiency is more common in the elderly, it's best to be on the lookout for adequate levels of B$_{12}$ to prevent dementia. Such dementia can often be reversed by injections of the vitamin, but this type of replacement has been found to work only when treatment begins early in the course of the dementia.
- **Calcium.** There is evidence that anticonvulsants directly affect bone cells and inhibit the transport of calcium. Therefore, a number of researchers recommend 1,500 mg of calcium supplementation a day in all patients at risk for osteoporosis.
- **Vitamin D.** Aging is associated with diminished levels of vitamin D, which increase the risk of bone fractures. Researchers recommend daily supplementation of 400 IU; patients who are at risk for vitamin D deficiency can benefit from taking between 400 and 800 IU per day.[5]

Stimulation

One of the major reasons for the decline in mental acuity and function seen in older people is a lack of mental and physical stimulation. After some people retire from jobs or after their children are grown, they have little to stimulate them.

Certainly, our memory slows and our physical bodies, subject to oxygen, gravity, and time, age. But mental stimulation is vital.

Playing cards, doing puzzles, writing letters, talking to people, playing bingo, playing and listening to music, taking adult education classes, and keeping up hobbies and interests play a major role in maintaining health. If your eyesight and reflexes aren't sufficiently keen, it's best to avoid driving. If no one is available to take you shopping or to the doctor, many communities provide senior bus service.

Light to moderate exercise also helps maintain good health. Walking, gardening, and swimming help keep muscles toned, reflexes good, and our bodies functioning, raising the seizure threshold. To avoid injury, use a cane or walker, if necessary.

As the population ages and the number of older patients with epilepsy increases, continuing research is needed to provide the safest and most effective treatments. Meanwhile, developing late-onset epilepsy doesn't doom us. "Probably because epilepsy hit me so late in life," says John Rawlings, a retired pharmacist who developed epilepsy at the age of seventy-five, "deep feelings of inadequacy and depression—including thoughts of suicide—marked the first eighteen months. In time, my depression became hopefulness and dejection was replaced by gladness. The day I laughed outright marked the end of suicidal thoughts. I have a great deal to be thankful for. I have a supportive family whom I love dearly. Few of us ever actually shake epilepsy. But we get better. I have learned that every action and thought must be played out in a positive, supportive manner. I cannot guess what the future might hold for me. I've come to believe that tomorrow could be a good day, perhaps the best of my life."

PART V

Creating a Supportive Environment

————————————————————

CHAPTER 17

Communicating and Nurturing

Happiness is a very powerful antiepileptic agent.
—Peter Fenwick, M.D., from his article "Influence
of Mind on Seizure Action" in *Epilepsy and Behavior*

People with epilepsy often feel lonely, unloved, unwanted. We some-times hate our bodies for betraying us. We fear intimacy, even though we crave it. We've often gotten unsympathetic, even unkind, messages from family, schoolmates, coworkers, or physicians who dealt long-lasting blows to our self-esteem. We often experience problems with dating, driving, employment, education, and insur-ance. Accepting our epilepsy but not allowing ourselves to be defined by it is a difficult, ongoing balancing act.

"It is important to be able to both connect with and distance yourself from one specific organ or condition," Dr. Fried once told me. "I would never have done the [experimental biofeedback study] if I thought that there is such a thing as an 'epileptic' versus some-one with seizures. For instance, you would say, 'I am disabled by such-and-such,' if you feel disabled. Otherwise, you would say, 'I have a disability, a grievous nuisance.' That way it is only a part of you. *To have* is not the same as *to be*."

Besides the self-anger, those of us with disabilities often feel we don't matter. And we all need to feel that we matter. It helps, I think, to ask, "What do I love to do? What do I feel drawn to?" That can be a guide. Many of us find purpose in work, in volunteer activities, and in our friends and families. Many people have an instinct to nurture, whether it's children, animals, or a garden. Since families can be hard to deal with, we often have to go outside of that circle for the support and encouragement we need. Therapy, as well as regular exercise and natural treatments, may help you feel closer to your body, to your inner self. Following intellectual pursuits with a sense of wonder and curiosity provides great relief from stressful thoughts and may even lead to solutions to problems.

Stigma

Stigmas were the signs used by the ancient Greeks to mark slaves, criminals, and other devalued persons. The centuries-old stigmas falsely linking epilepsy with demonic possession, retardation, and insanity linger. Epileptologist J. Kiffin Penry said flatly, "Epilepsy isn't treated very well." But some epilepsy researchers have distinguished between "enacted stigma," defined as instances of outright discrimination, and "felt stigma," defined as a fear of enacted stigma combined with more general shame about having epilepsy. These researchers suggest that "enacted stigma" has been overestimated in most studies and that "felt stigma" is a more important and devastating problem. But James Trostle, Ph.D., finds this to be a problematic position; it implies that people with epilepsy are themselves responsible for their difficulties. "The dominant culture of the United States values health, beauty, and control," says Trostle. "Epilepsy transgresses these values because a seizure can be interpreted as a sudden incarnation of unpredictability, physiologic dysfunction, and human frailty."[1] Diseases in general and chronic illnesses in particular can alter social relations: they turn wage earners into disabled people and family members into support networks.

Many persons with epilepsy feel stigmatized and ashamed. In one British survey, about a third of those who got married after their seizures began did not tell their prospective spouses about their epilepsy. Another third mentioned it, using words like "attacks," "dizzy spells," and other euphemisms.[2] More than half never told their employers they had epilepsy, and 18 percent of those who disclosed their epilepsy also reported job-related incidents that impaired their careers.

An Australian study indicated that levels of felt *and* enacted stigma are high among those with epilepsy. Of 160 epileptic outpatients, 58 percent complained that their social life was restricted, 39 percent felt their schooling was limited, and 44 percent believed their career was less successful than it would have been had they not had epilepsy.[3] A later Australian survey found that about 40 percent of fifty-one patients from a neurology clinic reported they had personally experienced job discrimination.

While 95 percent of respondents in one study believed most or all of their family knew about their seizures, 66 percent thought most or all of their friends knew, 55 percent thought most or all of their close coworkers knew, and 54 percent thought those usually around them knew. In addition, 35 percent were unlikely to disclose their epilepsy to a boss, 48 percent to a job interviewer, and 86 percent to a casual acquaintance. Overall, almost 40 percent of respondents gave low disclosure answers to four or more of the seven categories.[4]

Disclosure

Concerns about disclosure may be accentuated by embarrassed and protective family members, but, surprisingly, they may also be encouraged by some physicians. One physician reported that "at several epilepsy self-help meetings in the past few months, fully 80 percent of people attending have been warned by their neurologist to deny or cover up the diagnosis of epilepsy to deal with employers or insurance companies."[5] This attitude among so-called experts or authorities perpetuates the shame and fear. People whose epilepsy is mild or completely controlled can remain "in the closet" when it comes to driving and insurance. Yet there is some evidence that concealment itself causes additional problems, ranging from avoidance of social interactions to emotional damage.[6]

There are no hard and fast rules about whom you should tell. You should tell someone you have epilepsy only if you feel comfortable. However, in instances involving safety, such as operating heavy machinery or being around children, it's imperative that you mention your epilepsy. I would also suggest telling whomever you live with so that there's someone to call if there's ever an emergency.

Jeanne Carpenter, former president of the Epilepsy Foundation, in an article in *Epilepsy USA*, wrote:

> We have succeeded in getting epilepsy out of the closet and now we need to push it out onto the dance floor. It's easy to blame others for why epilepsy does not enjoy the level of public awareness or understanding, or what media people call "reach," that characterizes other disorders or diseases. But maybe we all should recognize that each of us with epilepsy can advance public understanding by realizing that

we have nothing to be ashamed of—that we sometimes perpetuate stigma with our own attitude and we should recognize that those around us need some education and explanation, not an apology.[7]

In my own life, I've found it easier and easier to say, "I have epilepsy." When I am open about it, it gives the other person the opportunity to ask questions. It also shows people that it's not something to be ashamed of. Frequently, when I say I have epilepsy, a person will say, "Oh, I take medication, too." It is one way people open up to each other, through our vulnerabilities.

Journalist Steve Fishman, author of *Bomb in the Brain*, developed seizures after a brain hemorrhage. In an article titled "Brainstorm," he wrote:

> Sometimes I gave up my cover. At first my voice trembled, like I'd been caught doing something wrong. But my new acquaintances didn't bolt. Moreover, and this was bizarre, epilepsy gave me access to people in a way I hadn't had before. One new friend said, 'I never tell this to anyone but I've been sick, too.' She was a recovering alcoholic.[8]

Emotions

The possibility of unpredictable seizures, worries about the reactions of other people, possible lifestyle limitations, and economic hardships often experienced by people with epilepsy compound the stressful nature of the disorder. So it is not surprising that emotional difficulties are most often cited by adults with epilepsy as being the single greatest problem they encounter. Problems with depression, learned helplessness, and general emotional distress are common in people with epilepsy.[9] A number of studies have found that adults with epilepsy are especially prone to significant problems with depression and general emotional distress.

Barbara Young, M.Ed., L.P.C., a Portland, Oregon, counselor, believes that for people with epilepsy, depression is strictly physiological. According to Young, depression and anxiety are the direct result of having seizures, and some doctors are beginning to investigate the problems of anxiety and depression as part of the epilepsy—not as side psychiatric symptoms.

Seattle nutritionist Jerri Spalding Fredin agrees:

> Dr. Janet Keller Phelps, who wrote a book on alcoholism based on her personal experiences, believed that most alcoholics experienced depression because of their abnormal metabolism of glucose. And I think down the road we will find documentation to link abnormal glucose metabolism not only to seizures but also to the depressions experienced by patients with seizures.

This connection could help to explain why so many of us with epilepsy also have hypoglycemia, or low blood sugar.

Bruce Hermann, Ph.D., believes that depression often goes unrecognized by patients and doctors. "People sometimes don't know they have depression," he says. "Or if they do, they just 'tough it out.' Or there may be limited access to treatment, a stigma regarding depression as mental illness, or lack of health insurance. And doctors have limited training regarding mental-health issues." He adds that tendencies toward depression run in families. So if a person has an innate vulnerability to depression, he or she may not cope as well with stressful life events (like seizures) as someone who doesn't have such a tendency.[10] Because untreated depression can lead to suicide, it's important that it be identified and treated. (Suicide rates among those with epilepsy are estimated to be four times higher than the general population.)

"Epileptic seizures should not be thought of as arising randomly," says Peter Fenwick, M.D., a British epileptologist and psychiatrist who has conducted numerous studies of the effect of emotions on seizure activity. He adds:

> Patients should be helped to understand that their seizures are intimately related to how they feel, what they are doing, and what they are thinking. . . . A complete treatment of epilepsy involves not just the giving of drugs but also teaching the patient about brain function, and the way their feelings, thinking, and behavior all can be used in the control of their seizures.[11]

And experts agree that stress is the main trigger of seizures. Carolyn Myss, a medical intuitive, has developed her intuition to do intuitive diagnosis, perceiving the source of illness through a person's energy. In her book *The Creation of Health*, she writes:

> In spite of the out-of-control nature of a seizure, my sense is that epileptic seizures frequently are "irrational" control mechanisms. They are a form of releasing emotion that a person is incapable of expressing directly or consciously. This is not meant as an unsympathetic evaluation of epilepsy; rather it is an interpretation of "seizures" that indicates a person is overwhelmed by intense emotions and is unable to cope through normal channels of expression.[12]

Support

Epilepsy is complex, involving more than just the seizures. A number of researchers believe that a major factor in human illness is the suppression of emotions. For example, Roger Dafter, a psychiatrist and associate director of the Mind-Body Medicine Group at UCLA Medical Center, argues that emotions traditionally considered negative actually can have positive biomedical properties. "Because turbulent emotions heat up the system, they can help to counter illnesses such as cancer," he explains. "In reality, you need emotions to help you survive."[13] Dafter based his research on recent studies indicating that cancer patients who express emotions such as antagonism and rage have better clinical outcomes than patients who behave "nicely."

These findings have a great deal of practical application for those of us with epilepsy. Many of us benefit greatly from therapies ranging from counseling to Jungian analysis to dance and art therapy. Dr. Fenwick mentions a forty-two-year-old woman who had been having generalized tonic-clonic seizures since she was sixteen. She also said she had feelings of déjà vu, sometimes associated with feelings of guilt. Her therapist helped her to deal with her guilt, and she described therapy as "the most powerful anticonvulsant" she had ever been given[14] (although, strictly speaking, she wasn't being given it, she was giving it to herself).

In another study, a group of Scottish patients with epilepsy received short-term psychological treatment without a change in medication. They experienced a significant reduction in their weekly seizure rate. Support groups, such as group meetings held by local affiliates of the Epilepsy Foundation or local epilepsy societies, can be very helpful. Hospitals, which host many support groups, may offer one for those with epilepsy. Some large companies sponsor groups for their employees, as well.

Because people shine when they are doing something they enjoy and are helping someone else, volunteering is a wonderful way to boost self-esteem while erasing feelings of isolation. There's also no need to fear being rejected because you're involved in activities in which you're needed. You're also likely to find others with common interests and values.

But we can't adequately nurture others if we don't adequately nurture ourselves. This is especially true of women, who tend to put others' needs ahead of their own. A sense of humor does wonders, transforming stressful situations into stress busters, emotionally and physically. When you are laughing, your body cleanses itself of stress.

"Research shows," says Dr. Christiane Northrup, "that the brain and organs in the body communicate with one another through chemical messengers called neuropeptides. Emotions and thoughts cause the brain to release neuropeptides, which attach to receptor sites throughout the body—meaning that our entire physical being is affected by our emotions."[15] Or, as my acupuncturist says, "Negative thoughts are poison to the body."

Sexuality

Ask a hundred people what they find really sexy, and you're bound to get a hundred different answers. That's because sex appeal is far easier to talk about than to define. Everyone, after all, is a passionate, complex sexual being with particular notions of what's sexy.

However, as a culture, we have more restrictive cultural notions of sexuality and sex appeal. We tend to view sexuality in terms of genital sensation and gratification, thereby ignoring whole areas of sensual delight. And we tend to equate sex appeal with current standards of physical beauty, reinforced by movies, television, and magazines, with men looking like athletes or rock stars and women having large breasts and small hips, as though love occurs only between two attractive people.

Even more restrictively, many people consider any kind of physical disability unattractive, even ugly. Lurking beneath this point of view is an even more troubling one: that it's somehow unseemly for disabled people to be concerned with attractiveness or with satisfying their sexual needs. It's as though pleasure and passion belong only to the physically attractive, or at least to those considered physically "normal."

It's no surprise, then, that people with disabilities often feel ashamed of their bodies and their sexuality. As Barbara Waxman, former disability project director for Los Angeles Planned Parenthood, says, "I don't see a message [coming from the culture] that good things can happen—like pleasure, intimacy, a greater understanding of ourselves, a love of our bodies."[16] She sees few, if any, positive models of sexuality and virtually no social acknowledgment that people with disabilities are sexual beings.

A poor body image alone can lead people with disabilities, or anyone else, for that matter, to think less of themselves. J. Kevin Thompson, Ph.D., an associate professor at the University of South Florida, says, "Obsessing over your physical shortcomings drains you of energy that could better serve you as the fuel for creativity, productivity, and self-realization." And this kind of energy and sense of self is really the basis of a healthy sexuality. As therapist Steven Handwerker, Ph.D., puts it, "Sex is an attitude. Doing what fulfills you is sexy. Developing your intellect is sexy. Thinking for yourself is sexy. Touch is sexy. Loving and accepting your body is sexy." Dr. Handwerker adds, "Caring about yourself is the most powerful drawing force. Because you're communicating from your heart and not draining somebody else with your expectations."

Undeniably, it can be difficult to accept a body that we feel can let us down at any time, perhaps even in moments of intimacy. Professional counseling and support groups are two ways to help understand and resolve the fear of a seizure during sexual activity. Discussing any fears you have with your partner, perhaps even practicing relaxation techniques together, can go a long way toward relieving anxiety and building intimacy.

Being loving and creative is an integral part of a healthy life. As writer Shakti Gawain states in her book *Creative Visualization*: "Our sexual energy comes from the same universal source as other energy. It is merely one way in which universal energy moves. through us and draws us to the experiences we need for our learning, healing and enjoyment."

Dogs: Helping People Be Independent

Dogs are proving once more that they are our best friends. Recent anecdotal studies have shown the apparent ability of some dogs to detect impending seizures in their owners. In effect, these dogs are serving as seizure early warning systems. (Cats, and even pet iguanas, have also reportedly assisted their owners who've had seizures.)

What Do They Do?

A seizure-alert dog has the ability to warn a person of an impending seizure moments or even hours before the person has clinical signs of a seizure. For example, Annie, a woman whose seizure activity caused her muscles to jerk suddenly without warning, often fell down during a seizure. Her Labrador retriever, Homer, would bark a warning, giving her time to sit down before the seizure occurred. Having this warning system in place meant Annie could go about her daily life without sustaining injury from a severe fall. Another woman, who has complex partial seizures, says her dog has stopped her before she crossed a street, thus preventing her from having a seizure in traffic.

How Do Dogs Know?

Interestingly, dogs do not have to be taught how to be seizure alert. There are two distinct phases of learned behavior in the dog. First, the dog recognizes that a seizure is going to occur. Then the dog physically reacts, by barking, licking its owner's face, acting restless, or some other sign.

"The theory widely accepted is that the dogs can pick up on chemical and electrical changes in the body," says Nicole McBride of Assistance Dogs International, in Cochranville, Pennsylvania. "Some people think that the dogs are alerted by slight changes in a person's body language or behavior before a seizure. Others think that the dog detects very subtle changes in a person's body odor. Whatever the mechanism, it's an ability that the dog exhibits immediately or develops over time while in contact with a person who has seizures. Many people who have seizures report seizure-alerting behavior in their dogs before a seizure. Or sometimes a dog doesn't 'predict' the seizure but stays by a person during the seizure and afterward. One man, who has seizures in his sleep, said if his wife wasn't around, 'I still knew not to stand and get up out of bed and possibly fall over because our dog would be at my bedside with a very worried look to identify that I had a seizure.'"

What Training Is Needed?

Seizure alerting is a behavior that a dog may already possess or it may have seizure-alerting potential. A good trainer encourages the alerting behavior after the dog alerts or shows the potential to alert. (Be skeptical of trainers who rely on pinch collars, chokers, or other devices to "control" the dog.) Due to lack of funding for research, all evidence so far has been anecdotal. Lacking scientific proof, it appears that a dog's perception of an oncoming seizure is not a behavior that can be trained in the conventional sense. It can only be identified and encouraged.

Ruby Joyce, who runs Sheppy's Disability Dogs in Westbrook, Maine, says she uses dogs' herding instinct. For example, one teenager would walk aimlessly before he dropped into a tonic-clonic seizure. "For him," Joyce says, "the dog needs to train to herd in circles to keep him out of streets or dangerous areas." She also trains her dogs to break falls. A large dog can take forty to fifty pounds off the impact of a fall by wiggling under a person and thereby possibly saving the person from injury.

"Prior to displaying the ability to alert to seizures," says Sue Miller of the Prison Pet Partnership Program in Gig Harbor, Washington, "these dogs have been so in tune with their person that they seem to know if the person is feeling happy, sad, or angry." (In this remarkable program, female inmates train dogs to assist the disabled as therapy or service dogs.)

Even if a dog isn't able to detect oncoming seizures, there are numerous benefits to having the dog with you. It can be taught to stay with a person throughout a seizure, and its familiar presence can comfort a person coming out of a seizure. Or the dog can be trained to bark or even activate an alarm when a person has a seizure. Since numerous studies indicate that animals help lower our stress levels and stress is a major seizure trigger, it's also possible that the presence of a loving animal can lower stress and potentially reduce seizure frequency. Joyce says that a number of clients whom she had trained dogs for have had fewer seizures.

For some, having the dog is a lifesaver. "It's the first time some people have ever gone out," says Joyce. "One woman finally enrolled in college, taking her dog with her every day." Still, Joyce is quick to point out that there's no guarantee. "And, in any case, we don't know if it will be a long-term benefit."

Like dogs for the visually impaired, seizure-alert dogs can be legally brought into schools, restaurants, and other public buildings. "A lot of people with epilepsy feel closed out, that others are insensitive to their condition," Joyce explains. "But as one woman said to me, 'I can look into my dog's eyes and I can tell he understands.'"

Epilepsy, by its very nature, remains surrounded by uncertainty. How our epilepsy impacts relationships with other humans, with social institutions, and with the communities in which we live profoundly affects our physical and mental health. We need to examine the difficulties we face and take full advantage of available resources for support and guidance.

CHAPTER 18

The World of Work
Being Competent and Conscientious

> *I realized I could no longer try to fit into a job's require-*
> *ments. I would have to match a job with my specific needs*
> *and abilities. The world of work would now have to meet*
> *me on my terms.*
>
> —Katinka Neuhof, who has cerebral palsy, from
> her article "Storming Castles"

It's been estimated that half of all people with epilepsy are under-employed or unemployed. One study of people with epilepsy indicated they formed a reasonably well educated group: 56 percent had high school diplomas, 38 percent had earned some college credits, and 15 percent had completed college degrees. Yet, 25 percent were unemployed—64 percent of these people believed they were unemployed as a direct result of their epilepsy.[1] This is a waste of human potential. We all need to feel useful, to feel there's a purpose to our lives, and many of us find this in the work we do.

The centuries-long discrimination that closed opportunities for people with disabilities is evaporating, so that few occupations are closed to us. We also have the law on our side. The Americans with Disabilities Act (ADA), passed by Congress in 1991, makes it illegal to discriminate against all disabilities, including "hidden" disabilities. It also requires employers to make "reasonable accommodations" for employees with disabilities.

Cases of job discrimination had been so numerous in the past that a special program for people with epilepsy was established in 1976 by the U.S. Department of Labor and the Epilepsy Foundation. The study that precipitated the program had shown that epilepsy ranked the lowest of all handicaps from which employers were willing to employ and that only 2 percent of persons with epilepsy were served by state vocational rehabilitation programs.

Most of employers' fears are unfounded. The majority of people with epilepsy never have seizures at work, our number of job-related accidents is lower, and we don't take more sick leave. One Dutch study comparing the general health status of patients with epilepsy with the general population found that those with epilepsy had more psychosocial problems and used health-care resources more often but weren't absent more from work or school and didn't have more problems at work.[2]

Exceptions

Generally, whether a person needs to be seizure free for any particular period of time depends on the actual job. For most jobs, a person's seizure history will not prohibit him or her from doing the work or from being considered qualified. However, people whose seizures are characterized by impaired consciousness, convulsions, or periods of disorientation may be excluded from jobs involving exposure to toxic chemicals or hot surfaces and operation of heavy machinery or motor vehicles because impairment of consciousness could cause injury to themselves or others.

Self-Doubt

While it's important to get the skills and training needed for a particular occupation, the biggest obstacle people with epilepsy face in attaining a job is self-doubt. Researchers who conducted the Dutch study mentioned above also found that people with epilepsy showed problems regarding self-confidence. Having seizures makes us doubt ourselves and our capabilities, and the fears of our families and friends often perpetuate this doubt.

On a personal note, after I graduated from college, my mother wanted me to get a secure, safe job with an insurance company or the government, with a regular salary, health benefits that covered visits to the neurologist's office, medical tests, and so forth, and a pension. Instead, I worked in a museum and wrote articles and short stories in my free time. When my first short story was published, my friends' mothers were more excited over my accomplishment than my own mother. I know she loved me, but she worried about me constantly, and, above all, she wanted me to be safe. Her own sense of security came from doing only what was expected of her. I was timid enough, but her discouragement gave me the feeling that I'd somehow disappointed her; if she had encouraged me, it would have made a big difference in how avidly I followed my dreams. I've learned that by setting goals, developing my inner resources, and networking, I spend less time waiting for others' validation and more time doing what I feel is best for myself.

The Epilepsy Foundation estimates that almost 80 percent of people with epilepsy can work "competitively"; that is, they can compete with others for jobs, and not just government-supported jobs or affirmative action jobs. Most people with epilepsy will never have a seizure at work. Still, we often have difficulty obtaining jobs suitable to our skills and interests. The Epilepsy Foundation operates a national employment assistance program, Employment Plus, to help those with epilepsy gain appropriate social skills (how to prepare for an interview, for example), assistance in putting together a resume, and job-hunting techniques.

For many of us with disabilities, home-based employment may be most suitable, especially since we often have difficulty obtaining jobs that match our skills and interests. Working at home also allows for flexibility in setting schedules and workload. With today's technology, the job opportunities are endless, from telemarketer to market researcher to freelance artist. And, of course, it solves the problem of transportation. Freelance writer Bill Clayton wrote: "In my first job out of college, I hitchhiked to work each day. In a suit. Rain or shine. Cold and snow . . . Odd behavior makes you a social suspect, so rides came infrequently, which meant I had to leave hours earlier than if I drove."[3]

Americans with Disabilities Act

Employers with fifteen or more employees are required to comply with the Americans with Disabilities Act (ADA). This legislation requires an employer to focus on ability and performance, not disability or medical issues. The ADA protects people with both hidden and open disabilities in an effort to somewhat level the playing field so that they will be seriously considered for employment. The ADA prohibits discrimination on the basis of disability in all phases of the job-application process, including application forms, interviews, testing, and medical examinations.

Previously, job applications often contained questions about disabilities or illness; if an applicant answered "yes," he or she might never get called for an interview. Though it is not actually illegal for an employer to ask what your religion or nationality is, it is illegal to ask if you have a disability. You are under no obligation to disclose your epilepsy, or any disability, before a position of employment is offered.[4]

Employers may not make inquiries of any kind regarding an individual's disability unless the inquiry is specifically related to the applicant's ability to perform a job-related function. For example, if someone applied for a job at a health-food store, a legitimate question would be, "Can you lift a twenty-pound sack of potatoes?" An employer may ask about a job applicant's ability, reliability, work-attendance history, training, and experience—all questions that presumably are being asked of everyone.

An employer may ask someone who is obviously disabled—in a wheelchair, say—"Can you perform this function?" and even ask how he or she would perform a certain job duty; for example, "How would you teach rowing?" If the applicant is able to answer these questions satisfactorily, stating that he or she would be able to perform all the necessary functions of a job, the employer would have no legal right to give the job to someone else based on the presence of a disability.

Disclosure

Although you're not bound to disclose your epilepsy before an offer of employment has been made, you might want to mention it. William Wolpert, Ed.D., former director of vocational services at the Epilepsy Institute in New York City, offers the following suggestions:

- You may choose to defer your disclosure during the interview until your competence for the prospective job has been discussed. You might want to say something like, "I want to be forthright and honest with you, since I don't wish to withhold information. I occasionally have seizures, but they do not interfere with my work routine." You can mention that in prior jobs your seizures have not hampered your capability or productivity.

- You might mention the type of seizures you have and how you manage them, whether you are taking medication and so forth. Make it easy for the employer to discuss any concerns, saying, for example, "I'm open to any questions and concerns you might have." If he or she is interested in more information about epilepsy, such as literature or films, you can contact the Epilepsy Foundation, which does presentations to companies to educate employees about epilepsy.
- Emphasize that having epilepsy would in no way affect your high degree of motivation and commitment to the position, should it be offered.

People who do reveal a disability during an interview and then don't get the job often wonder, "Was it epilepsy that kept me from getting the job?" For this reason you may decide not to disclose your epilepsy during the interview and wait until you have been offered the job. If you accept, you may want to disclose your epilepsy just before or upon starting work. You can say, "I want to be forthright with you. I sometimes have seizures, but they do not interfere with my work routine or my motivation."

Once a job has been offered, an employer—who presumably has found the applicant qualified—is allowed to ask questions related to disabilities and to do medical examinations of employees if they are job related and consistent with business necessity.

Reasonable Accommodation

Most people with epilepsy need no special job accommodations. However, sometimes flexibility in scheduling or an accommodation to ensure safe job performance is necessary.

Although no one is required to disclose a disability before an offer of employment is made, it might be a good idea to mention it, especially to discuss "reasonable accommodation." These are modifications or adjustments to the work environment or to the manner or circumstances under which the position is customarily done that enable a qualified individual with a disability to perform the essential functions of that job or modifications or adjustments that enable an employee with a disability to enjoy benefits and privileges (including pay, tenure, promotion, transfer, layoff). For a person with seizures, such accommodations might include but aren't limited to:

- Assigning regular shifts rather than rotation or split shifts for someone whose seizure activity increases with irregular schedules and fatigue
- Allowing for flexibility in scheduling for those who need to use public transportation
- Giving an employee who is photosensitive a computer monitor with a nonflicker, low-glare screen
- Assigning an employee with epilepsy to work on machines equipped with "deadman" switches that turn off the machine automatically in case of an accident or seizure
- Restructuring a job slightly so that the inability to do one or two tasks won't prevent a person with epilepsy from doing the job. For example, someone with epilepsy who works as a bookkeeper may not be able to take a deposit to the bank because he or she doesn't have a driver's license; another employee can take on this task.
- Allowing an employee with epilepsy to take medication at required times, or working with a doctor to revise the medication schedule if it interferes with work

The ADA requires an employer to make reasonable accommodation unless it creates undue hardship for the employer, which may include significant difficulty or expense incurred by the employer. A study by the Job Accommodation Network, a free technical service sponsored by the President's Committee on Employment of People with Disabilities, found that the cost of most accommodations is about two hundred dollars.[5]

Although the ADA requires employers to make reasonable accommodation, there is no set deadline for providing such accommodation. If an employer is dragging his or her feet, it is helpful to keep track of how many times you asked for the accommodations, what you were told, and what, if any, action was taken. You can remind your employer that he or she is subject to jury trial and punitive damages for refusing to try to come across with the reasonable accommodations.

A Seizure on the Job

Although you probably will never have a seizure at work, you should inform your supervisor and coworkers what should be done in case of a seizure on the job. Posting first aid measures near your work station or in an easily accessible area makes it easier for coworkers to respond as well.

If you do have a seizure, says Dr. Wolpert, take time to orient yourself before you speak. When you feel alert, don't apologize; assure everyone that you are all right and you just need a few moments to get yourself together and you'll get back to work. Thank people who helped you. If some people did something inappropriate—such as trying to stuff tissues in your mouth because they were afraid you might swallow your tongue—let them know you appreciate their concern and explain what sort of help would be more appropriate should you have another seizure. It can also be helpful to discuss what happened with those who witnessed the seizure. You may feel awkward and embarrassed, but acting as though nothing happened can make you feel more isolated and leave their questions about epilepsy unanswered.

If people express doubt that you can perform your job, make a careful examination of your work performance including how well you collaborate with other employees. Show them that the facts are on your side.

Jay, who has absence seizures, had difficulties with the pressure of working as a cashier in a very large hardware store. He finally informed his boss that he had absence seizures and asked to work in another part of the store. They denied his request and fired him. With the help of his disability support group, he sued them. "It wasn't that they couldn't accommodate someone with epilepsy," Jay says. "They actually have a good record in hiring people in wheel-chairs and older people." Fortunately, he got his job back several months later, along with several thousand dollars in reimbursement for lost wages.

The ADA has recently been challenged in the Supreme Court. "Some attorneys are predicting that there will be little or no impact; others are predicting major problems," says Alta Hancock, employ-ment director at the Epilepsy Foundation of Oregon. "My guess is that many employers will provide the accommodations without dis-pute. Some employers may test it. As with any change in law, it will be tested in the courts."

For now, the ADA remains a valuable tool for those of us with epilepsy. Having labor laws on our side helps us find work we care about. We can retire the myths that people who have epilepsy are lazy, unconscientious, have more accidents, and are less productive than the general public.

CHAPTER 19

How to Choose and Work with a Health-Care Practitioner

You've got to advocate for yourself. No one's going to kick the doctor's butt but you.

—CONNIE BERGLUND, WHO HAS EPILEPSY

One thing just about everyone who's sought treatment for epilepsy agrees on is that often there is a poor doctor-patient relationship: Doctors who want to treat the symptoms, not the patient. Doctors who don't explain treatment. Who don't listen. Who immediately dismiss nonpharmaceutical treatments as quackery. Such doctors are becoming less common—due in large part, I think, to increasing education about epilepsy and patients' advocating for their own health.

In general, many people aren't satisfied with the medical care they receive. What may distinguish the problems that people with epilepsy have with their doctors is that, because of the intimacy of a neurological disorder and the lack of knowledge about that disorder, there's a bit more potential for friction. James Trostle, Ph.D., writes in his article "Social Aspects of Epilepsy":

> There is some evidence that patients with epilepsy prefer to know more information about their condition and its treatment than neurologists usually offer. . . . Studies suggest that interaction between patients and physicians can be filled with unexpressed and unacknowledged conflict.[1]

He adds that neurologists seem to be far more likely than patients to believe that physicians should be responsible for making health-care decisions.

The shame and helplessness we often feel make it easier for us to slip into patterns of passivity and helplessness, believing our health to be utterly dependent on a doctor. As John Robbins, author of *Diet for a New America*, says, "We struggle as a culture to get over the idea that M.D. stands for 'Medical Deity.'" Many of the neurologists I've seen behaved like sergeants giving orders. Like a lot of people with epilepsy, I've been passive with neurologists. Shame and feelings of helplessness contributed to this, as well as the complexity of neurology—what do I know about the brain compared to someone who spent eight years in medical school and dissected cadavers? But I think I also wanted to avoid conflict. When I finally became more assertive, I found a neurologist who listened to me, one who admitted the value of alternative therapies.

Knowledge Leads to Healing

An essential element of enhancing our healing response is having a sense of control over our health, as opposed to a sense of helplessness. Knowledge does that. In the words of Ernest Rosenberg, M.S.: "Knowledge boosts faith in a positive outcome."

We can be more informed about epilepsy by doing our own research: reading books and articles, talking to experts, and searching the Internet. Searching websites for health information is rapidly becoming more popular (even doctors search for and exchange information). Many good sites have links to sources such as research journals or professional societies. One of the wonderful things about the Internet is its international aspect, making it easy to find information from all over the world, information that might not be available in the country in which the Web searcher is located. Most of the health information on the Internet is presented from the standard conservative medical viewpoint. Websites that offer alternative information are still in the minority. One word of caution: While there is a great deal of solid health information on the Internet, there is also a lot of misinformation. Just because something is on a website doesn't mean it's accurate or true!

If you decide to do an Internet search, be sure to try different search engines (Yahoo, Netscape, Google, Excite, and so on) and try different key words. Many libraries offer classes on researching the Internet. Even if you don't own a computer, free access to the Internet is available at most public and university libraries. Reference librarians will be happy to assist you.

Being Prepared

In addition to being passive, many patients aren't always honest with their physicians. One large poll indicated that 50 percent of those with epilepsy said they didn't report seizures to their doctor and 55 percent said they do not report medication side effects.[2] Another study of people with epilepsy found that 70 percent alternated their medication dosage on their own; 15 percent said they had discontinued it completely. Physicians refer to this as noncompliance, but, more important, issues of side effects aren't being examined.

It seems that what patients want and what physicians want regarding seizure control are sometimes at odds. Doctors view seizures largely in terms of severity and frequency. But some patients have occasional seizures that don't affect their ability to work or study or their general quality of life. Or they may find that medication makes them sleepy, lethargic, interferes with their creativity or sex life. In any case, they may want little or no medication. On the other hand, their doctor wants them to be totally seizure free, which for some can be achieved only with medication. The point is, instead of sneaking medication changes, we need to decide what we need or want from our medical treatment and tell that to our doctors. "The psychological and social dimension of epilepsy is a realm where doctors receive the least education and people often experience the greatest problems," says Orrin Devinsky, M.D. "Physicians need to understand—and patients need to make them understand—that each patient is different."

In fairness to doctors, they go through rigorous training that emphasizes disease and mechanistic ways to treat illness. "There is absolutely no teaching about healing in the medical curriculum today," says Andrew Weil, M.D. "I think this is the single greatest defect in standard medicine."[3] Marti Ann Schwartz, author of *Listen to Me, Doctor*, says, "Doctors aren't gods; nurses aren't angels. Most doctors are uncomfortable with the belief that doctors have all the answers. They would prefer, they told me, to emphasize the teamwork that comes from working with informed patients."[4]

If you have epilepsy, you need to speak to a doctor who is supportive of your right to do everything you possibly can to prevent seizures and make yourself healthy. We are health-care consumers, after all, and if we don't feel we're getting good treatment from a

Questions to Ask Your Doctor

1. What is the diagnosis?
2. What treatment are you planning?
3. How will this treatment deal with the cause of the seizures?
4. When might I expect treatment to work?
5. What can I do to improve my health (or the health of my child)?
6. What reading material can you recommend?
7. What other options might you try if this treatment plan doesn't work?
8. Are you willing to work with an alternative health practitioner (nutritionist, chiropractor, or herbalist, for example)?

health-care practitioner, we should go to another. And another. Until we find one we feel comfortable with and can work with effectively. Rather than relying on doctors as saviors, says Dr. Christiane Northrup, we need to consider them as partners, using individual knowledge about our bodies to make our own informed decisions.

It's important to evaluate how comfortable you feel with the health-care practitioner and staff, if you feel confident of their professional skills, if they involve you in decision making, and if they adequately answer your questions (which you should write down before an appointment.) Ultimately, you need to be satisfied with the treatment and care you are receiving. Some very good physicians who are holistically oriented and open to alternative treatments and patient collaboration don't necessarily call themselves holistic; and some physicians who call themselves holistic aren't. The more research you do, the more likely you are to know when a particular doctor (or any health-care practitioner) is right for you.

The Alternative Approach

Alternative approaches have one thing in common: they honor the entire body. They aim to support and strengthen the body's powerful healing forces. They work with the body to unleash its healing abilities. David M. Eisenberg, M.D., director of the Center for Alternative Medicine at Beth Israel Deaconess Medical Center in Boston, recommends that a patient ask the alternative-care provider the following questions about a proposed treatment:

- How will it help me?
- What is your experience with similar patients?
- How many treatments will it take before I experience improvement?
- How much will treatment cost?
- Are you willing to talk with my medical doctor about my case?

Dr. Eisenberg strongly believes that all providers must be willing to communicate openly with one another and with their patients about these issues. When an alternative provider has been chosen and a care plan devised—such as biofeedback treatments or nutritional therapy—he proposes that the patient and medical doctor meet again before the alternative treatment begins to review the proposed protocol for safety, toxicity, and potential conflicts with the conventional treatment and prescription drugs.[5]

Dr. Eisenberg stresses that decision making should be a process shared by the patient with conventional and alternative providers alike. Furthermore, he says, doctors need to "give their patients permission" to tell their stories about alternative treatments.

While not all alternative therapies appeal to everyone, we need to decide what we value and what we don't. We can do this by listening to our bodies, reading, and learning what our bodies and minds need. Modern medicine certainly offers much of value. Yet, because conventional medicine relies heavily on pharmaceuticals, which merely suppress symptoms, it can be of great value to consult health practitioners of alternative treatments. Ideally, they can work with your doctor. Complementary medicine, the collaboration between conventional and alternative providers, is in everyone's best interest. The patient's participation in this health-care process will ensure that it becomes their standard of care.

CHAPTER 20

Summing Up

Epilepsy, like any handicap, like being unemployed or picked last on the playground, is not so much a question of what you can and can't do, but of how you feel about those facts.

—STEVE FISHMAN, FROM HIS ARTICLE "BRAINSTORM" IN *Hippocrates*

My doctor refers to epilepsy as "a black box," a metaphor that captures its complexity, uncertainty, and the fear surrounding seizures. But it seems to me to be like a *matryoshka* (those Russian dolls-within-a-doll)—there's always more to be revealed.

Since I was diagnosed with epilepsy when I was twenty-one, the question of *why* has remained with me, an undercurrent that has crested into wave after wave of questions. It wasn't until after I began looking at how I treated my body, how my thoughts affected my mind and my body, specifically my seizures, that I was drawn to alternative treatments. And I stopped wondering, "How can I get rid of my epilepsy?" and started wondering, "How can I understand it?"

Says John Robbins in the magazine *EarthSave International*:

When we are taught to repress symptoms with no attempt to understand the needs these symptoms represent, our experience of ourselves becomes distant. We sense our bodies not as sources of self-awareness and guides to our healing needs, but as enigmas that must be analyzed and explained to us by experts. We easily become bewildered and lose trust in ourselves.[1]

Since I began having seizures, I've had to expend a lot more care and attention on my body than others who take good health for granted. I've never been satisfied with my body, never thought I could do anything about it; it just existed. And when I began having seizures, that dissatisfaction was compounded by anger and contempt. Drugs took me further away from myself. But when I began changing the nourishment I took, the way I breathed, the way I moved, and even my expectations of myself, it was amazing to me that my body responded. I, not a doctor, was giving myself health and a feeling of well-being. Whereas medication made me feel like a stranger to my own body, alternative treatments brought me closer to myself. In *The Ice Age*, a novel by Margaret Drabble, a man reflects on his heart and the extra care and awareness he's had to give it since he had a heart attack. "Now that he was growing accustomed to its presence," Drabble writes, "he was learning to feel affection for it." Like that character, I've come to cherish my body, to be aware of her needs.

I hope this book helps readers to better understand their bodies and how to help prevent seizures by healing their bodies, not merely suppressing symptoms. Whether you try nutritional supplements, biofeedback, psychotherapy, or yoga, it's extremely important to be gentle with yourself. John O'Donoghue, an Irish priest, poet, and scholar, says that when he works with people who are ill, he has them conduct a conversation with the part of their body that is ill, to talk to it as though it were a partner, to thank it for all it has done despite all it has suffered and whatever pressure people might have put on it. We need to be grateful for our bodies and how well they take care of us, especially considering that for most of us the seizures account for a tiny fraction of our lives.

I'm sure there are alternative treatments not included here that people have found helpful. As research into alternative medicine increases, I look forward to learning about more treatments, especially those studying the mind-body connection—to me, one of the most fascinating aspects of epilepsy. Neither the mind nor the body exists separately; they are always working together. I think we have a far better chance of understanding them if we are gentle with ourselves, if we seek natural ways to respond to illness.

I tend to fall into problems more easily than I create solutions, so I'm especially grateful to all the people who have helped me focus on solutions to my seizures, not on the problems seizures cause. That includes health professionals, but also it includes so many people with epilepsy whom I've encountered. They've taught me a lot. They helped me say "epilepsy" without faltering. I hope all of us with epilepsy can learn to speak up, while listening to the voice within ourselves.

RESOURCES

Information about epilepsy and general health is available in numerous places. Listed are excellent sources of information—books, organizations, and websites—that I've found useful. They concern epilepsy as well as general health. (Addresses and telephone numbers may be subject to change.)

Books

Blaylock, Russell. *Excitotoxins: The Taste That Kills.* Santa Fe, NM: Health Press, 1994.

DesMaisons, Kathleen. *Potatoes Not Prozac.* New York: Simon & Schuster, 1999.

Fadiman, Anne. *The Spirit Catches You and You Fall Down.* New York: Farrar, Straus & Giroux, 1997.

Fishman, Steve. *Bomb in the Brain.* New York: Scribner's, 1988.

Green, Bernard. *Getting Over Getting High.* New York: William Morrow & Co., 1984 (out of print).

Lechtenberg, Richard. *Epilepsy and the Family.* Cambridge, MA: Harvard University Press, 1984.

Leppik, Ilo, M.D. *Contemporary Diagnosis and Management of the Patient with Epilepsy*, Fourth Edition. Newtown, PA: Handbooks in Health Care, 1998.

Manheim, C. and D. Lavett. *Craniosacral Therapy and Somato-emotional Release: The Self-Healing Body.* Thorofare, NJ: Slack, Inc., 1992.

Marshall, Fiona. *Epilepsy: The Natural Way.* Boston: Element Books, 1998.

Penfield, Wilder, and H. Jasper. *Epilepsy and the Functional Anatomy of the Brain.* Boston: Little, Brown, 1956.

Reiter, Joel, M.D., et al. *Taking Control of Your Epilepsy: A Workbook for Patients and Professionals, The Basics.* Santa Rosa, CA, 1987. (Available by mail-order from Andrews-Reiter Epilepsy Project, Inc., 550 Doyle Park Drive, Santa Rosa, CA 95405.)

Richard, Adrienne, and Joel Reiter, M.D. *Epilepsy: A New Approach*, Second Edition. New York: Walker Books, 1995.

Schachter, Steven, M.D., et al., eds. *The Brainstorms Family: Epilepsy on Our Terms.* Philadelphia: Lippincott-Raven Publishers, 1996.

Stoler, Diane R., Ed.D., and Barbara A. Hill, M.S. *Coping with Mild Traumatic Brain Injury.* Garden City Park, NY: Avery Publishing Group, 1998.

Upledger, John. *Your Inner Physician and You: Craniosacral Therapy.* North Atlantic Books, 1992.

Waltz, Mitzi. *Partial Seizures.* Sebastopol, CA: O'Reilly Publishers, 2001.

Breath and Meditation

Benson, Herbert, M.D. *The Relaxation Response.* New York: Outlet Books, Inc., 1993.

Borysenko, Joan. *Minding the Body, Mending the Mind.* Reading, MA: Addison Wesley, 1987.

Cohen, Kenneth S. *The Way of Qigong: The Art and Science of Chinese Energy Healing.* New York: Ballantine Books, 1997.

Fried, Robert, Ph.D. *The Breath Connection.* New York: Plenum Press, 1990.

Fried, Robert, Ph.D. *The Psychology and Physiology of Breathing in Behavioral Medicine, Clinical Psychology, and Psychiatry.* New York: Plenum Press, 1993.

Hendricks, Gay. *Conscious Breathing.* New York: Bantam Books, 1995.

LeShan, Lawrence. *How to Meditate.* Boston: Little, Brown, 1974.

Herbs

Hoffman, David. *The New Holistic Herbal.* Boston: Element Books, 1997.

Mowrey, Daniel B. *Herbal Tonic Therapies.* New Canaan, CT: Keats, 1993.

Mowrey, Daniel B. *Scientific Validation of Herbal Medicine.* New Canaan, CT: Keats, 1990.

Weed, Susun. *Healing Wise.* Woodstock, NY: Ash Tree Publishing, 1989.

Nutrition

Appleton, Nancy. *Lick the Sugar Habit.* Garden City Park, NJ: Avery Publishing, 1996.

Balch, James, M.D., and Phyllis Balch. *Prescription for Nutritional Healing.* Garden City Park, NY: Avery Publishing Group, 2000.

Blaylock, Russell, M.D. *Excitotoxins: The Taste That Kills.* Santa Fe, NM: Health Press, 1997.

Brake, Dennis, and Cynthia Brake. *The Ketogenic Cookbook.* Pennycorner Press, 1997. (Do not attempt this diet without medical supervision.)

Freeman, John, M.D. *The Epilepsy Diet Treatment: An Introduction to the Ketogenic Diet,* Second Edition. New York: Demos Publishers, 1996.

Graedon, Joe, and Teresa Graedon, Ph.D. *Dangerous Drug Interactions: The People's Pharmacy Guide.* New York: St. Martin's Paperbacks, 1999.

Null, Gary, Ph.D. *Get Healthy Now!* New York: Seven Stories Press, 1999.

PDR (Physicians' Desk Reference). Medical Economics Company, 1998.

Philpott, William, M.D. *Brain Allergies.* New Canaan, CT: Keats, 1985.

Roberts, H. J., M.D. *Aspartame/NutraSweet: Is It Safe?* Philadelphia: Charles Press, 1990.

Roth, June. *The Food/Depression Connection: A Cookbook for Controlling Allergy-Based Mood Swing.* Chicago: Contemporary Books, 1978.

Smith, Lendon, M.D. *Feed Your Body Right.* New York: M. Evans, 1993.

Weintraub, Skye, N.D. *Allergies and Holistic Healing.* Pleasant Grove, UT: Woodland Publishing, 1997.

Articles

Andrews, Donna, Ph.D., and W. H. Schonfeld. "Predictive Factors Controlling Seizures Using a Behavioral Approach." *Seizure*, vol. 1 (1992): 111–116.

Efron, Robert, M.D. "The Conditioned Inhibition of Uncinate Fits," *Brain* (1957): 251–261.

Fenwick, Peter, M.D. "The Relationship Between Mind, Brain, and Seizures," *Epilepsia*, 33 (Supplement 6): S1–S6, 1992.

Fishman, Steve. "Brainstorm." *Hippocrates* (September/October 1988): 67–74.

Fredin, Jerri Spalding. "New Hope for People with Epilepsy," *Journal of Orthomolecular Medicine*, vol. 4, no. 4 (1989): 193–203.

Hippocrates. "On the Sacred Disease," *Hippocrates and Galen: The Great Books*, vol. 10. Chicago: Encyclopedia Britannica, 185.

Richard, Adrienne. "Integrating Mind, Brain, Body, and Spirit in Treating Epilepsy," *Advances: The Journal of Mind-Body Health* (Fall 1992): 7–19.

Wood, Rebecca. "Baking Without Wheat," *Natural Health* (January/February 2000): 104–107, 148–150.

Publications

Epilepsy Wellness Newsletter
1462 West Fifth Avenue
Eugene, OR 97402
(541) 686-9125
www.epilepsywellness.com

Published quarterly, this newsletter reports on the growing evidence—scientific and anecdotal—indicating the substantial benefits of alternative treatments for people with epilepsy. Such treatments can be used in lieu of or in conjunction with prescribed medication.

Natural Health magazine
70 Lincoln Street, Fifth Floor
Boston, MA 02111
www.naturalhealthmag.com

Alternative Health magazine
1650 Tiburon Boulevard
Tiburon, CA 94920
(800) 515-4325
www.alternativemedicine.com

Organizations

Epilepsy Foundation
4351 Garden City Drive
Landover, MD 20785
(800) 332-1000
www.efa.org

The Epilepsy Foundation provides information on educational, social, legal, and treatment issues for people with seizure disorders. It also publishes educational materials and offers books, videos, and pamphlets through its catalog. Its website offers state-by-state guidelines for driver's licenses. Epilepsy Foundation affiliates in metropolitan areas around the country offer employment and educational programs, counseling, and support groups. The Foundation holds an annual conference, open to the public.

Victoria Epilepsy and Parkinson's Centre Society
813 Darvin Avenue
Victoria, BC V8X 2X7
(250) 475-6677
www.vepc.bc.ca

Victoria Epilepsy and Parkinson's Centre (VEPC) provides information, videos, and pamphlets and conducts epilepsy support groups. A newsletter is published four times a year.

Epilepsy Canada
1470 Peel Street, Suite 745
Montreal, QC H3A 1T1
(514) 845-7855
www.epilepsy.ca

Epilepsy Canada offers pamphlets and videos and publishes a newletter twice a year, in English and French.

The Charlie Foundation to Cure Pediatric Epilepsy
1223 Wilshire Boulevard
Santa Monica, CA 90403
(800) 367-5386

The Charlie Foundation provides information regarding the ketogenic diet. A free video that describes the diet can be obtained by calling or writing the foundation.

Keto Klub
61557 Miami Meadows Court
South Bend, IN 46614
(219) 299-3438

This organization is a support group for parents whose children are on the ketogenic diet.

Well Mind Association (WMA)
4649 Sunnyside Avenue North, Room 344
Seattle, WA 98103
(206) 547-6167

This nonprofit organization is dedicated to helping victims of brain dysfunction and environmental sensitivities. WMA publishes a quarterly newsletter.

Seizure-Alert Dogs
Prison Pet Partnership Program
9601 Bujacich Road
P.O. Box 17
Gig Harbor, Washington 98335-0017
(206) 858-4240

This organization trains seizure-alert dogs and helps people with epilepsy obtain dogs.

Employment

Job Accommodation Network (JAN)
www.jan.wvu.edu

This is an international toll-free consulting service, providing information on job accommodations and the employability of people with disabilities. JAN is a service of the President's Committee on Employment of People with Disabilities: www50.pcepd.gov/pcepd.

Women's Issues

Women and Epilepsy Initiative
Epilepsy Foundation
4351 Garden City Drive
Landover, MD 20785
(301) 459-3700, ext. 623

Women and Epilepsy Initiative currently supports research targeting women and girls, provides information on how epilepsy affects women, advocates improved medical care, and promotes a greater understanding of how epilepsy affects females.

Antiepileptic Drug Pregnancy Registry
(888) 233-2334
www.aedpregnancyregistry.org

This pregnancy registry has been established by an independent scientific advisory group and financed by five pharmaceutical companies that manufacture anticonvulsants.

Alternative Therapy

The legality of practicing certain forms of alternative therapies varies from state to state. Some states require licensing in particular therapies, while others do not. In some states, a patient must be referred by a physician. In others, they are considered primary health-care providers. The following organizations provide information, along with the names of practitioners in your area.

Acupuncture

www.acupuncture.com

Acupressure

Acupressure Institute
(510) 845-1059

Alexander Technique

American Society for the Alexander Technique
P.O. Box 3992
Champaign, IL 61826
(800) 473-0620
www.alexandertech.org

Aromatherapy

National Association for Holistic Aromatherapy
(314) 963-2071
www.naha.org

Ayurvedic Medicine

Ayurvedic Institute
(505) 291-9698
www.ayurveda.com

Biofeedback

Association for Applied Psychophysiology and Biofeedback
(800) 477-8892
www.aapb.org

Chiropractic

American Chiropractic Association
1701 Clarendon Boulevard
Arlington, VA 22209
(800) 986-4636
www.amerchiro.org

Craniosacral Therapy

Cranial Academy
3500 Depaw Boulevard
Indianapolis, IN 46268
(317) 879-0713

Upledger Institute
11211 Prosperity Farms Road
Palm Beach Gardens, FL 33410
(407) 622-4206

SORSI (S.O.T.)
P.O. Box 8245
Prairie Village, KS 66208
(913) 649-3475

Herbs

Herb Research Foundation
1007 Pearl Street, Suite 200
Boulder, CO 80302
(800) 748-2617
www.herbs.org

This organization conducts herbal research and provides information about herbs and their uses.

American Holistic Medical Association
6728 Old McLean Village Drive
McLean, VA 22101
(703) 556-9728

Contact this organization for referrals to a physician knowledgeable about herbs.

Homeopathy

International Foundation for Homeopathy
2366 Eastlake Avenue, Suite 301
Seattle, WA 98102
(206) 324-8230
www.homeopathic.org

Massage

American Massage Therapy Association
820 Davis Street, Suite 100
Evanston, IL 60201
(312) 761-2682

Naturopathy

American Association of Naturopathic Physicians
(206) 298-0125
www.naturopathic.org/FindND.html

Osteopathy

American Academy of Osteopathy
(317) 879-1881, ext. 17
www.am-osteo-assn.org

Osteopathic Center for Children
College of Osteopathic Medicine of the Pacific
4135 Fifty-fourth Place
San Diego, CA 92105-2303
(619) 583-7611

Reflexology

International Institute of Reflexology
(727) 343-4811

Rolfing

Rolf Institute of Structural Integration
(303) 449-5903
www.rolf.org

Traditional Chinese Medicine

American Association of Oriental Medicine
(888) 500-7999
www.aaom.org

Yoga

International Association of Yoga Therapists
(415) 332-2478

Websites

Epilepsy Connection: http://www.epilepsy-connect.org/home/index
.shtml. This website, written by people with epilepsy, offers a wide
variety of information about seizures and social issues, as well as
services to individuals and employers.

Alternative Therapies: http://www.healthonline.com/alther
.htm

Choices: www.choices.com. This website was founded by the Citizens for Alternative Health Care. CAHC believes that integrative health care encourages the use of the best alternative and allopathic treatments.

The website of Andrew Weil, M.D., who is probably the most prominent doctor advocating alternative health treatments, includes a section on epilepsy: www.drweil.com

National Institutes of Health, Office of Alternative Medicine: http://nccam.nih.gov

NOTES ———————————————————————————

Chapter One

1. Rilke, Rainer Maria. (1934) *Letters to a Poet.* New York: W.W. Norton.

Chapter Two

1. Epilepsy Foundation of America, Landover, Maryland: www.efa.org.
2. Sander, Ley, and Pam Thompson. (1989) *Epilepsy: A Practical Guide to Coping.* Wiltshire: The Crowood Press, 73.
3. Richard, Adrienne and Joel Reiter, M.D. (1989) *Epilepsy: A New Approach.* New York: Prentice Hall, 106.
4. Hippocrates. "On the Sacred Disease." *Hippocrates and Galen: The Great Books*, vol. 10. Chicago: Encyclopaedia Britannica, 154.
5. Lopez, Barry. (1978) *Of Wolves and Men.* New York: Charles Scribner's Sons, 236.
6. Fishman, Steve. (1988) "Brainstorm: My Career as an Epileptic," *Hippocrates* (October), 67.
7. Bettman, Otto. (1974) *The Good Old Days—They Were Terrible.* New York: Random House, 149.

8. Fishman, Op. Cit., 68.

9. Trostle, James. (1980) "Social Aspects of Epilepsy," *Epilepsia* (43), 39–45.

10. Fadiman, Anne. (1997) *The Spirit Catches You and You Fall Down: A Hmong Child, Her American Doctors, and the Collision of Two Cultures.* New York: Farrar, Straus & Giroux.

11. Kleinman, Arthur. (1980) *Patients and Healers in the Context of Culture.* Berkeley, CA: University of California Press.

Chapter Three

1. Theodore, William. *Neurology*, January 1999.

2. Wade, Nicholas. (1999) "Brain Growth Continues into Adolescence," *New York Times* (October 15), 1A.

3. Aven, Allan B. (1979) Selected Letters in Response to Advertisements Requesting Information About Non-Medicinal Approaches to Coping with Epilepsy. Epilepsy in the Urban Environment Project, Center for Urban Affairs and Policy Research, Northwestern University, 5.

4. Laber, Emily. (1998) "Fried Couch Potatoes," *The Sciences* (March-April), 12.

5. Harding, G., and P. Jeavons. (1994) *Photosensitive Epilepsy.* London: MacKeith Press.

6. Kosta, Louise. (1990) "Electromagnetic Fields: Unanswered Questions," *The Human Ecologist* (winter), 1–6.

7. Takahashi, T., and Y. Tsukahara. (1992) "Usefulness of Blue Sunglasses in Photosensitive Epilepsy," *Epilepsia*, 33 (3), 517–521.

8. Ottman, Ruth, and Richard Lipton. (1995) "Relationship Between Epilepsy and Migraines," *Neurology* (February).

9. Nilsson, L., et al. (1999) "Risk Factors for Sudden Unexpected Death in Epilepsy: A Case-Control Study," *Lancet* (March 13), 888–893.

10. Mendez, M. F., et al. (1986) "Depression in Epilepsy," *Archives of Neurology* (August), 766–770.

11. *Epilepsy Wellness Newsletter.* Fall 1999, 7.

12. Donker, G. A., et al. (1997) "Epilepsy Patients: Health Status and Medical Consumption," *Journal of Neurology* (June), 365–370.

Chapter Four

1. Leppik, Ilo. (1998) *Contemporary Diagnosis and Management of the Patient with Epilepsy*, Fourth Edition. Newtown, PA: Handbooks in Health Care, 50.

2. Morello, Gaetano. (1996) "Treating Epilepsy Effectively," *American Journal of Natural Medicine* (October), 14–20.

3. Marshall, Fiona. (1998) *The Natural Way: Epilepsy*. Boston: Element Books, 30.

4. Sugarman, G. I. (1984) *Epilepsy Handbook: A Guide to Understanding Seizure Disorders*. New York: Mosby.

5. Leppik, Op. Cit., 86.

6. Ibid., 75.

7. Dahllof, G. (1993) "Periodontal Condition of Epileptic Adults Treated Long-Term with Phenytoin or Carbamazepine," *Epilepsia* (September-October), 960–964.

8. Drew, H. U., et al. (1987) "Effect of Folate on Phenytoin Hyperplasia," *Journal of Clinical Perodontology* (14), 350.

9. Burton Goldberg Group, comp. (1997) *Alternative Medicine*. Puyallup, WA: Future Medicine Publishing, 917.

10. *FDA Consumer.* (1997) "Food and Drug Adminstration Approves NeuroCybernetic Prosthesis System," *FDA Consumer* (November-December), 4.

11. Freeman, J. M., et al. (1998) "The Efficacy of the Ketogenic Diet: A Prospective Evaluation of Intervention in 150 Children," *Pediatrics* (December), 1358–1363.

12. *Eastside (WA) Journal*, February 8, 1999.

13. Petry, Judith J. (1997) "Supplements for Successful Surgery," *Association of Operating Room Nurses Journal* (June), 81–85.

14. Fried, Robert. (1993) "Breathing Training for the Self-Regulation of Alveolar CO_2 in the Behavior Control of Idiopathic Epileptic Seizures," *Neurobehavioral Treatment of Epilepsy*, David Mostofsky and Ynvge Loyning, eds. Hillsdale, NJ: Lawrence Erlbaum Associates, 21.

15. *Newsweek* (1998) "Americans Are Turning to Alternative Medicine," *Newsweek* (November 23), 68.

16. Weil, Andrew. (1998) "Critique of *New England Journal of Medicine*'s Attack on Alternative Medicine," *Self-Healing* (November), 40–43.

Chapter Five

1. Morello, Gaetano. (1996) "Treating Epilepsy Effectively," *American Journal of Natural Medicine* (October), 14–20.

2. *Lancet*, June 14, 1997.

3. Marshall, Fiona. (1998) *The Natural Way: Epilepsy*. Boston: Element Books, 79.

4. Braly, James, M.D. (1999) "Detecting Hidden Food Allergies," *Alternative Medicine Digest* (issue 24), 79–84.

5. Author interview.

6. Reichelt, K. L., et al. (1990) "Gluten, Milk Proteins, and Autism: Dietary Intervention Effects on Behavior and Peptide Secretion," *Journal of Applied Nutrition*, 42 (1), 1–11.

7. Haavik, S., et al. (1979) "Effects of the Feingold Diet on Seizures and Hyperactivity: A Single-Subject Analysis," *Journal of Behavioral Medicine*, 2 (4), 365–374.

8. Weintraub, Skye, N.D. (1997) *Allergies and Holistic Healing*. Pleasant Grove, Utah: Woodland Publishing, 18.

9. Ibid.

10. Fredericks, Carlton. (1982) *Nutrition Guide for the Prevention and Cure of Common Ailments and Diseases.* New York: Simon & Schuster, 59–60.

11. Egger, J., et al. "Oligoantigenic Diet Treatment of Children with Epilepsy and Migraine," *Journal of Pediatrics* (114), 51–58.

12. Atkins, Robert C. (1998) *Dr. Atkins' Vita-Nutrient Solution: Nature's Answers to Drugs.* New York: Simon & Schuster.

13. Fredin, Jerri Spalding. (1989) "New Hope for People with Epilepsy," *Journal of Orthomolecular Medicine*, vol. 4, no. 4, 193–203.

14. Reading, Chris, and Meillon, R. S. (1988) *The Family Tree Connection.* New Canaan, CT: Keats.

Chapter Six

1. Brown, H. Morrow. (1985) *The Allergy & Asthma Reference Book.* London: Harper & Row, 84.

2. Kraus, G. L., and E. Niedermeyer. (1991) "Electroencephalogram and Seizures in Chronic Alcoholism," *Electroencephalography and Clinical Neurophysiology*, vol. 78, 97–104.

3. Appleton, Nancy. (1988) *Lick the Sugar Habit.* Garden City Park, NY: Avery Publishing, 112.

4. Alvarez, Walter. (1976) *Help Your Doctor Help You.* Berkeley, CA: Celestial Arts.

5. Fredin, Jerri Spalding. (1989) "New Hope for People with Epilepsy." *Journal of Orthomolecular Medicine*, vol. 4, no. 4, 193–203.

6. Gittleman, Louise Ann. (1996) *Super Nutrition for Men.* New York: M. Evans, 164.

7. Bond, Charles S. (1898) "A Consideration of Four Cases of Epilepsy with Reference to Cause," *Journal of the American Medical Association* (August 19), 670.

8. Editorial, "Epilepsy and Other Diseases Due to Albumin Starvation and Sugar Poisoning," *Medical Review of Books*, July 1910.

9. Blaylock, Russell. (1997) *Excitotoxins: The Taste That Kills*. Santa Fe: Health Press, 15.

10. Smith, Lendon. (1993) *Feed Your Body Right*. New York: M. Evans, 188.

11. Allen, R. B. (1983) "Nutritional Aspects of Epilepsy." *International Clinical Nutrition Review* (3), 3–9.

12. Morello, Gaetano. (1996) "Treating Epilepsy Effectively," *American Journal of Natural Medicine* (October), 14–20.

13. Fredin, Op. Cit.

14. Blaylock, Op. Cit., 158.

15. Olney, J. W. (1988) "Excitotoxic Food Additives: Functional Teratological Aspects," *Progressive Brain Research* (18), 283–294.

16. Gold, Mark. (1995) "The Bitter Truth About Artificial Sweeteners," *Nexus* (December-January), 71–75.

17. Blaylock, Op. Cit, 158.

18. Smith, Op. Cit.

Chapter Seven

1. Smith, Lendon. (1993) *Feed Your Body Right*. New York: M. Evans, 188–189.

2. Morello, Gaetano. (1996) "Treating Epilepsy Effectively," *American Journal of Natural Medicine* (October), 14–20.

3. Crowell, G. F., and E. S. Roach. (1983) "Pyridoxine-Dependent Seizures," *American Family Physician* (27), 183–187.

4. Ibid.

5. Nakazawa, M., et al. (1983) "High-Dose Vitamin B_6 Therapy for Infantile Spasms: The Effect and Adverse Reactions," *Brain Development* (5), 1937.

6. Graedon, Joe, and Teresa Graedon. (1996) *Deadly Drug Interactions: The People's Pharmacy Guide.* New York: St. Martin's Press.

7. Hoffer, A. (1962) *Niacin Therapy in Psychiatry.* Springfield, IL: Charles C. Thomas.

8. Krause, K. H., et al. "B Vitamins in Epileptic," *Bibliotheca Nutricion y Dieta* (38), 154–167.

9. Flodin, N. W. (1988) *Pharmacology of Micronutrients.* New York: Alan R. Liss.

10. Christiansen, C. (1974) "Anticonvulsant Action of Vitamin D," *British Medical Journal* (ii), 2589.

11. Ogunmekan, A. (1988) "Is There a Role for Vitamin E Therapy in Epilepsy?" *International Clinical Nutrition Review*, 8(1), 50–52.

12. Ogunmekan, A., and P. A. Hwang. (1989) "A Randomized, Double-Blind, Placebo-Controlled Clinical Trial of D-alpha-tocopheryl Acetate (Vitamin E) as Add-On Therapy, for Epilepsy in Children," *Epilepsia* (30), 84–89.

13. Pfeiffer, Carl. *Mental and Elemental Nutrients.* New Canaan, CT: Keats, 278, 402–408.

14. Smith, Op. Cit.

15. Pfieffer, Carl, and S. LaMola. (1983) "Zinc and Manganese in the Schizophrenics." *Journal of Orthomolecular Psychiatry* (12), 215–234.

16. Tanaka, Y. (1977) "Low Manganese Level May Trigger Epilepsy," *Journal of the American Medical Association* (238), 1805.

17. Barbeau, A., and J. Donaldson. (1974) "Zinc, Taurine, and Epilepsy," *Archives of Neurology* (30), 52–58.

18. Sterman, M. B., et al. (1988) "Zinc and Seizure Mechanisms," *Nutritional Modulation of Neural Function.* J. Morley, M. B. Sterman, and J. Walsh, eds. New York: Academic Press, 307–315.

19. Konig, S., et al. (1994) "Severe Hepatoxicity During Valproate Therapy: An Update and Report of Eight New Fatalities," *Epilepsia* (35), 1005–1015.

20. Roach, E. S., and L. Carlin. (1982) "N, N-dimethylglycine for Epilepsy," *New England Journal of Medicine* (307), 1081–1082.

21. Birdsall, Timothy C., N.D. (1998) "Therapeutic Applications of Taurine," *Alternative Medicine Review*, 3 (2), 128–136.

22. Durell, L., et al. (1983) *Clinical Neuropharmacology*, vol. 6, (March), 37.

23. Atkins, Robert C. (1998) *Dr. Atkins' Vita-Nutrient Solution: Nature's Answers to Drugs.* New York: Simon & Schuster.

Chapter Eight

1. Freeman, John M. (1997) *Seizures and Epilepsy in Childhood: A Guide for Parents.* Baltimore: Johns Hopkins University Press, 152.

2. *Tufts University Health and Nutrition Letter* (1997) "A Diet for Epilepsy Provides New Hope," *Tufts University Health and Nutrition Letter* (June).

3. Freeman, John M., et al. (1998) "The Efficacy of the Ketogenic Diet: A Prospective Evaluation of Intervention in 150 Children," *Pediatrics* (December), 1358.

4. Freeman, John M. (1997) *Seizures and Epilepsy in Childhood: A Guide for Parents.* Baltimore: Johns Hopkins University Press.

5. Ibid., 151.

Chapter Nine

1. Murphy, Patricia. (1997) "Healing with Herbs," *Epilepsy Wellness Newsletter* (summer), 3.

2. Sifton, David, ed. (1999) *The Physicians Desk Reference Family Guide to Natural Medicines and Healing Therapies.* New York: Three Rivers, 1204.

3. Foster, Steve. (1999) "Black Cohosh: A Literature Review," *Herbalgram* (winter), 47–48.

4. Sifton, Op. Cit., 122.

5. *Natural Health* magazine, September-October, 1994.

6. Marshall, Fiona. *Epilepsy: The Natural Way.* Boston: Element Books, 53–54.

7. *New York Times,* July 20, 1997.

8. *Townsend Letter for Doctors,* June 1995, 86.

9. Morello, Gaetano. (1996) "Treating Epilepsy Effectively," *American Journal of Natural Medicine* (October), 14–20.

Chapter Ten

1. Richard, Adrienne, and Joel Reiter. (1990) *Epilepsy: A New Approach.* New York: Prentice Hall, 214.

2. Murphy, Patricia. (2000) "Biofeedback: Reprogramming Your Brain," *Epilepsy Wellness Newsletter* (summer), 3.

3. Robbins, Jim. (1996) "Reprogramming the Brain," *New Age Journal* (March-April), 138.

4. Fried, Robert, Mary Fox, and Richard Carlton. (1990) "Effect of Diaphragmatic Respiration with End-Tidal CO_2 Biofeedback on Respiration, EEG, and Seizure Frequency in Idiopathic Epilepsy," *Annals of the New York Academy of Sciences,* 67–96.

5. Author interview, January 23, 1996.

6. Fried, Robert. (1993) "Breathing Training for the Self-Regulation of Alveolar CO_2 in the Behavioral Control of Idiopathic Epileptic Seizures," *Neurobehavioral Treatment of Epilepsy,* David Mostofsky and Ynvge Loyning, eds. Hillsdale, NJ: Lawrence Erlbaum Associates, 23.

7. Ibid.

8. Andrews, Donna, and W. H. Schonfeld. (1992) "Predictive Factors Controlling Seizures Using a Behavioral Approach," *Seizure*, vol 1., 111–116.

9. Richard and Reiter, Op Cit, 144.

10. Whitman, S., et al. (1989) "Progressive Relaxation for Seizure Reduction," a publication of the Center for Urban Affairs and Policy Research, Northwestern University, Evanston, Illinois.

11. Roth, David, et al. (1994) "Physical Exercise, Stressful Life Experience, and Depression in Adults with Epilepsy," *Epilepsia*, 35 (6), 1248–1255.

12. Nakken, K. O., et al. (1997) "Does Physical Exercise Influence the Occurrence of Epileptiform EEG Discharges in Children?" *Epilepsia*, 38 (3), 279–284.

13. Albrecht, H. (1986) "Endorphins, Sport, and Epilepsy: Getting Fit or Having One?" *New Zealand Medical Journal*, 99 (814), 915.

14. Liporace, J. D. (1997) "Women's Issues in Epilepsy," *Postgraduate Medicine* 102 (1), 123–127.

15. Cutts, Sandy. (1996) "Epilepsy Puts Cyclist on Road to Olympics," *Epilepsy USA* (September), 1.

16. Deepak, K. K., et al. (1994) "Meditation Improves Clinicoelectroencephalographic Measure in Drug-Resistant Epileptics," *Biofeedback and Self-Regulation*, vol. 19, no. 1.

17. (1996) *Indian Journal of Medical Research*, vol. 103, 165.

18. Folan, Lilias. (1998) "The Thirty-Second Stressbuster," *Country Living's Healthy Living* (February-March), 25.

19. Ibid.

20. Hughes, J. R., et al. (1998) "The 'Mozart Effect' on Epileptiform Activity," *Clinical Electroencephalography*, 29 (3), 109–119.

21. Hughes, J. R., J. J. Fino, and M. A. Melyn. (1999) "Is There a Chronic Change of the 'Mozart Effect' on Epileptiform Activity? A case study," *Clinical Electroencephalography*, 30 (2), 44–45.

22. Fenwick, Peter. (1991) "The Influence of Mind on Seizure Activity," *Epilepsy and Behavior*, 412.

23. Efron, Robert. (1957) "The Conditional Inhibition of Uncinate Fits," *Brain*, 251–261.

24. *Science News*. "Seizure Prelude Found by Chaos Calculation," (1993) *Science News* (May 23), 326.

25. Marshall, Fiona. (1999) *Epilepsy: The Natural Way*. Boston: Element Books, 29.

26. Null, Gary. (2000) *The Food-Mood-Body Connection*. New York: Seven Stories Press, 158.

27. Richard and Reiter, Op. Cit., 198.

Chapter Eleven

1. Klide, A. M., et al. (1987) "Acupuncture Therapy for the Treatment of Intractable Idiopathic Epilepsy in Five Dogs." *Acupuncture Electrotherapy Research*, 12(1), 71–74.

2. Lai, C. W., and Y. Lai. (1991) "History of Epilepsy in Chinese Traditional Medicine," *Epilepsia* (May-June), 289–302.

3. Alcantara, J. (1998) "Chiropractic Management of a Patient with Subluxations, Low Back Pain, and Epileptic Seizures," *Journal of Manipulative and Physiological Therapeutics*, 21 (6), 410–418.

4. Marshall, Fiona. (1998) *Epilepsy: The Natural Way*. Boston: Element Books, 68.

5. Author interview, July 20, 1999.

6. Marshall, Op. Cit., 86.

Chapter Twelve

1. Kosta, Louise. (1996) "The Environment and the Nervous System: Seizure Disorders—What Are They?" *The Human Ecologist* (spring), 9.

2. Gilbert, Mary, et al. (1989) "Pyrethroids and Enhanced Inhibition in the Hippocampus of the Rat," *Brain Research*, 477: 314–321.

3. Cox, C. (1996) "Herbicide Factsheet: Glufosinate," *Journal of Pesticide Reform* (winter), 5–19.

4. Singer, R. (1990) "Neurotoxicity and Environmental Illness," *The Human Ecologist* (winter), 15–17.

5. Kosta, Louise. (1996) "Seizures and Multiple Chemical Sensitivity: Is There a Connection?" *Human Ecologist* (spring), 10.

6. Wiles, R., and K. Davies. (1995) "Pesticides in Baby Food." Environmental Working Group and National Campaign for Pesticide Policy Reform, Washington, D.C.

7. Gurunathan, S., et al. (1998) "Accumulation of Chlorpyrifos on Residential Surfaces and Toys Accessible to Children," *Environmental Health Perspective* (106), 9–16.

8. Allen, R. B. (1983) "Nutritional Aspects of Epilepsy," *International Clinical Nutrition Review* (3), 3–9.

9. Mothers for Natural Law: www.safe-food.org.

10. *Healthy Living*, November 1999.

11. *USA Today*, June 29, 1999.

Chapter Thirteen

1. Shearer, A. (1999) "Seizures and Epilepsy in Childhood," *Exceptional Parent* (August), 64–66.

2. Ogunmekan, A., and P. A. Hwang (1990) "A Randomized, Double-Blind Placebo-Controlled Clinical Trial of Epilepsy in Children," *Epilepsia* (30), 1.

3. Marshall, Fiona. (1999) *Epilepsy: The Natural Way*. Boston: Element Books, 78.

4. Barnet, L. B. (1959) *Journal of Clinical Physiology* (1), 25.

5. Suplee, Curt. (2000) "Key Brain Growth Goes on into Teens: Study Disputes Old Assumptions," *The Washington Post* (March 9), A1.

6. Ibid.

7. Fredin, Jerri Spalding. (1989) "New Hope for People with Epilepsy," *Journal of Orthomolecular Medicine*, vol 4, no. 4., 193–203.

8. Smith, Philip. (1998) "The Teenager with Epilepsy Has Special Needs," *British Medical Journal* (October 10), 960.

9. Gross, Meir. (1979) "Incestuous Rape," *Journal of the American Orthopsychiatric Association*, 704–708.

10. Murray, J. A., and M. Haynes. (1996) "The Benevolent Overreaction: Nursing Assessment and Intervention in Families Coping with Seizure Disorder," *Journal of Neuroscience Nursing* (August), 100–105.

11. Ibid.

12. Kaufman, Pat. "Frustration: The Emotion Caregivers Know Too Well," *Take Care!*, newsletter of the National Family Caregivers Association, 10.

13. Schacter, C., et al., eds. (1996) *The Brainstorms Family: Epilepsy on Our Terms.* Philadelphia: Lippincott-Raven, 46.

14. Ibid, Foreword.

15. Lechtenberg, R. (1984) *Epilepsy and the Family.* Cambridge, MA: Harvard University Press.

16. Stalland, N., P. Osborne, and P. Shafer. (1998) "When the Parent Has Epilepsy," *Managing Seizure Disorders*, Nancy Santilli, ed. Philadelphia: Lippincott-Raven, 189–197.

17. Ibid.

Chapter Fourteen

1. Morrell, Martha. (1998) "Issues for Women with Epilepsy," *Western Journal of Medicine* (April), 266–270.

2. Mims, Janet. (1996) "Sexuality and Related Issues in the Preadolescent and Adolescent Female with Epilepsy," *Journal of Neuroscience Nursing* (April).

3. Herzog, A. G. "Progesterone Therapy for Women with Complex Partial and Secondary Generalized Seizures," *Neurology* (45), 1660–1662.

4. Morrell, Op. Cit.

5. Jensen, Eric, et al. (1990) "Sexual Dysfunction in Male and Female Patients with Epilepsy: A Study of 86 Outpatients," *Archives of Sexual Behavior*, vol. 19, no. 1, 1–14.

6. *Nutrition Almanac*, Second Edition. (1984) New York: McGraw-Hill.

7. Tallmadge, Alice. (1997) "Managing Menopause," *Eugene Weekly* (October 23), 23.

8. Foster, Steve. (1999) "Black Cohosh: A Literature Review," *Herbalgram* (winter), 48.

9. Cummings, S. R., et al. (1985) "Epidemiology of Osteoporosis and Osteoporotic Fractures," *Epidemiological Review* (47), 178.

10. Herzog, A., et al. (1986) "Reproductive Endocrine Disorders in Women with Partial Seizures of Temporal Lobe Origin," *Archives of Neurology*, vol. 43, no. 4, 341–346.

Chapter Fifteen

1. Pedley, T., and B. Mekdrum, eds. (1995) "Endocrine Aspects of Epilepsy in Men," *Recent Advances in Epilepsy*, vol. 6, 239–245.

2. Austin, J. K., et al. (1996) "Adjustment Issues in Persons with Epilepsy," *Managing Seizure Disorders*, N. Santilli, ed. Philadelphia: Lippincott-Raven, 211–225.

3. Taneja, N., et al. (1994) "Effect of Phenytoin on Semen," *Epilepsia* (January-February), 136–140.

4. Gallig, Katherine. (1999) "Sperm and Organic Produce," *Natural Health* (May), 31.

5. Jensen, Eric, et al. (1990) "Sexual Dysfunction in Male and Female Patients with Epilepsy: A Study of 86 Outpatients," *Archives of Sexual Behavior*, vol. 19, no. 1, 1–14.

6. Statistics from the Epilepsy Foundation of America.

7. *Lumina*. "Side Effects of Anticonvulsants," *Lumina* (publication of Epilepsy Canada), (autumn), 12.

Chapter Sixteen

1. National Cancer Institute SEER Program data.

2. Leppik, Ilo. (1998) *Contemporary Diagnosis and Management of the Patient with Epilepsy*, Fourth Edition. Newtown, PA: Handbooks in Health Care, 91.

3. Dreifuss, F. (1996) "Epilepsy in the Elderly," *Managing Seizure Disorders*, N. Santilli, ed. Philadelphia: Lippincott-Raven, 119–123.

4. Blaylock, Russell. (1997) *Excitotoxins: The Taste That Kills*. Santa Fe: Health Press, 189.

5. Valimaki, M. J., et al. (1994) "Bone Mineral Density Measured by Dual-Energy Absorption and Novel Markers of Bone Formation and Reabsorption in Patients on Antiepileptic Drugs," *Journal of Bone Mineral Research* (9), 631–637.

Chapter Seventeen

1. Trostle, James. (1986) "Social Aspects of Epilepsy," *Epilepsia*, 39–41.

2. Ibid.

3. Trostle, J., and V. E. Edwards. (1974) "Social Problems Confronting a Person with Epilepsy in Modern Society," *Proceedings of the Australian Association of Neurology* (11), 23–43.

4. Trostle, Op. Cit., 41.

5. Ibid.

6. Dell, J. (1986) "Social Dimensions of Epilepsy: Stigma and Response," *Psychopathology in Epilepsy*, S. Whitman and B. H. Hermann, eds. New York: Oxford University Press, 185–210.

7. Carpenter, Jeanne. (1999) "President's Message," *Epilepsy USA* (May), 12.

8. Fishman, Steve. "Brainstorm," *Hippocrates* (September-October), 67–74.

9. Roth, David, et al. (1994) "Physical Exercise, Stressful Life Experience, and Depression in Adults with Epilepsy," *Epilepsia*, 35 (6), 1248–1255.

10. Hermann, Bruce. What's New in Epilepsy? A speech given at the Epilepsy Foundation Annual Conference, August 1999.

11. Fenwick, Peter. (1992) "The Relationship Between Mind, Brain, and Seizures," *Epilepsia* 33 (Supplement 6), S1–S6.

12. Myss, Carolyn, and C. Norman Shealy. (1998) *The Creation of Health*. New York: Three Rivers Press, 227.

13. Finkelstein, Katherine Eban. (1988) "Research for Your Life: Investigating Your Own Health Care," *On the Issues* (spring), 38.

14. Fenwick, Op. Cit., 53.

15. Sullivan, Karin H. Interview with Dr. Christiane Northrup in *Vegetarian Times*, July 1995, 55–59.

16. Murphy, Patricia. "Epilepsy and Sexuality," *Epilepsy Wellness Newsletter* (winter), 5.

Chapter Eighteen

1. Fisher, R. S., et al. A Large Community-Based Survey of Quality of Life and Concerns of People with Epilepsy, Part 1. Presented at the American Epilepsy Society Annual Meeting, December 9, 1998.

2. Donker, G. A., et al. (1997) "Epilepsy Patients: Health Status and Medical Consumption," *Journal of Neurology*, 244(6), 365–370.

3. Clayton, Bill. (1999) "Seize the Day," *Hour Detroit Magazine* (March).

4. Mastroianni, P. (1995) "Pre-Offer vs. Post-Offer Inquiries: Equal Employment Opportunity Commission's (EEOC) Position," *In the Mainstream*, (May-June), 16–21.

5. Varnet, T. (1999) "On the Edge of Change," *Exceptional Parent*, (August), 25–31.

Chapter Nineteen

1. Trostle, James. (1986) "Social Aspects of Epilepsy," *Epilepsia*, 44.

2. Epilepsy Awareness Study, 1996. Conducted by the National Family Opinion Research, Inc.

3. Weil, Andrew. (1995) *Alternative & Complementary Therapies* (September-October).

4. Schwartz, M. A. (1996) *Listen to Me, Doctor*. Denver: Mac-Murray and Beck.

5. Eisenberg, David. Advising Patients Who Seek Alternative Therapy. Lecture at University of Washington, November 13, 1997.

Chapter Twenty

1. Robbins, John. (1996) "Reclaiming Our Health," *EarthSave International* (Fall), 2–7.

INDEX